image matters
FOR MEN

with colour**me**beautiful

Veronique Henderson
& Pat Henshaw

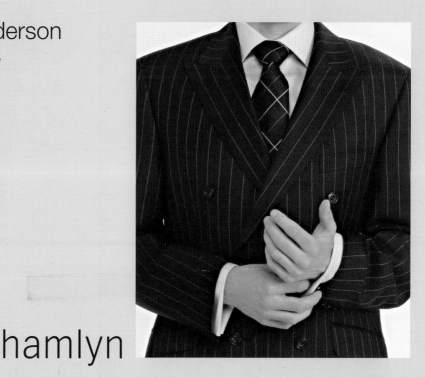

hamlyn

To Chris, David, Jim, John, Steve and Tom.

First published in Great Britain in 2006 by
Hamlyn, a division of Octopus Publishing Group Ltd
2–4 Heron Quays, London E14 4JP

Distributed in the United States and Canada by
Sterling Publishing Co., Inc.
387 Park Avenue South, New York, NY 10016-8810

ISBN-13: 978 0 600 61518 7
ISBN-10: 0 600 61518 9

A CIP catalogue record for this book
is available from the British Library

Printed and bound by Butler & Tanner, Frome

10 9 8 7 6 5 4 3 2 1

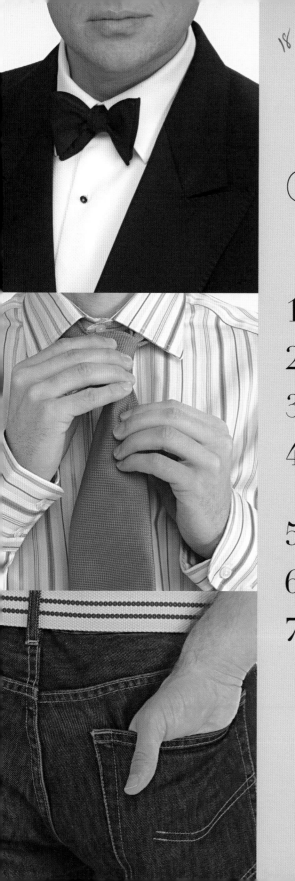

18

Contents

Introduction

We live in an age where we are surrounded by visual images – from huge billboards to pixellated photos on tiny mobile phones. In today's world it is no longer only the famous actor whose image is in public view, but that of every politician, businessman and sports personality. Quite apart from their actions and words, their clothes, their haircuts and even their footwear may be discussed at length in the media.

Why image matters

For all of us, whether we are public figures or not, managing our appearance is an important part of who we are. It makes a visual statement about our personality and our lifestyle, as well as indicating our abilities and confidence. In today's world, image really does matter.

> You have 30 seconds to make a first impression, which can last up to 15 years.

Thirty-second impact

Think how quick we are to judge people we meet on social or business occasions. Do you remember what they were saying? Do you recall the tone of their voice? Or do you remember what they wore?

Research by Professor Albert Mehrabian, in his book *Silent Messages*, first published in 1971, shows that 55 per cent of our behaviour and appearance and 38 per cent of the sound of our voice are remembered from the first 30 seconds of meeting someone, while only seven per cent of what we say will make any impact. So, like it or not, 93 per cent of how you come across has nothing to do with what you are saying.

Further research done with CEOs and HR executives shows that the three most important elements they consider when making a new appointment are:

✓ Communication skills (verbal and written).

✓ Personal image (grooming, manners and dress).

✓ Qualifications.

The upshot is that you should always think carefully about what you wear, for the simple reason that if you feel comfortable in your clothes, your body language will be more positive, your eye contact better and you will sound more confident.

Why buy this book?

This book, from the world's leading image consultancy **colour me beautiful**, provides you with the answers to all your wardrobe challenges – from deciding which tie to wear with a certain shirt for work or whether an 'occasion' calls for a suit or a jacket. It will give you the knowledge you need to create the look you want – and to enjoy doing so. You need to be your own man, to dress the way that makes you feel comfortable and to project the image you deserve.

Whatever your age and size, this book will lead you, step by step, towards recognizing the best colours for you to wear and the most appropriate styles of shirts, jackets, trousers and casual clothes for your build. There are guidelines to help you understand your personal look so you can develop a style that coordinates all the clothes in your wardrobe; you'll also find out what you should be looking for when buying clothes. In later chapters, there is guidance on what to wear for various occasions, what to pack for trips away from home and how to look after your clothes, as well as tips on skincare and determining the best hairstyle and choice of spectacles for your face shape.

The well-dressed man

The book will help you build on all the elements necessary to be the 'well-dressed man', as defined by **colour me beautiful** and its corporate division **cmb**corporate. You should wear clothes that:

✓ Complement your colouring.

✓ Balance your build, scale and proportions.

✓ Fit your personality.

✓ Are appropriate for the occasion, be it business or social.

✓ Are up to date.

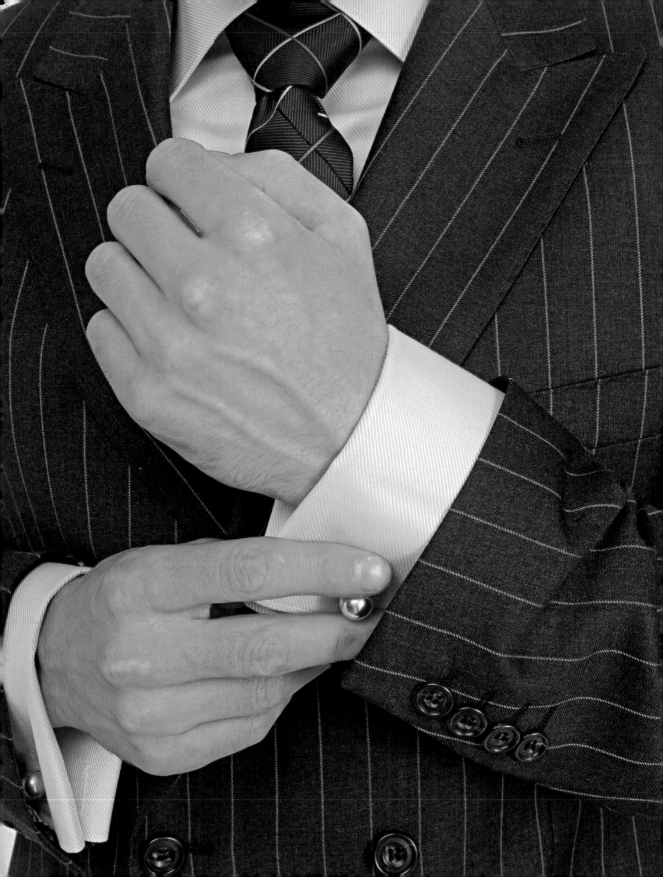

1

clothes make the man

What your clothes say about you

For most men, shopping for clothes brings no joy. They find there are too many choices, they don't have enough time for shopping and often have a general lack of interest in clothes. Although a shirt or sweater may not be the most exciting of Christmas or birthday presents, it often relieves the recipient of the need to shop for it.

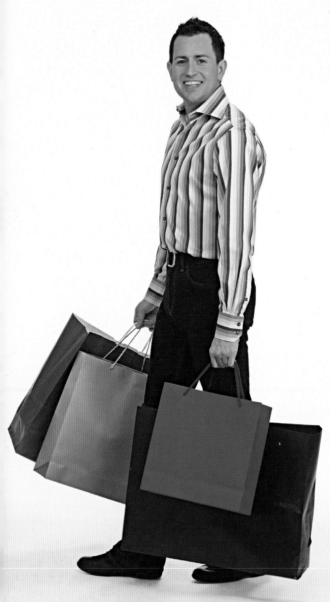

You and your clothes

Men often rely on a sister, mother or partner to help them make their clothes purchases, or even do their shopping for them. If you leave your choice of clothes to others, bear in mind that family intervention in your wardrobe may reflect how those close to you see you and wish to influence you, rather than how you wish to be perceived by the rest of the world. Your thoughtful grandmother, for example, may have spent hours knitting you that cardigan but the end result says more about her knitting skills than it should say about you.

Do any of the following statements reflect your attitude to clothes and dressing?

✓ You only buy clothes when necessary.

✓ Somebody else buys all your clothes.

✓ Your look is the same every day, including the weekend and evenings out.

✓ You always wear the same colours.

✓ You own only three pairs of shoes, including sports trainers.

✓ You only wear ties given to you as a present.

✓ You find grooming a chore.

If so, this book is for you. It may also be useful for anyone wanting to help and guide the man in their life towards a coordinated wardrobe with minimum effort.

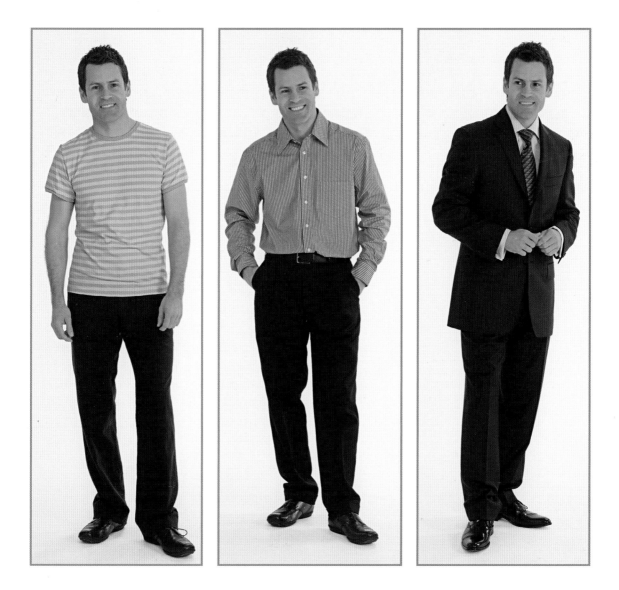

You'll find getting your look right for your age and the occasion is simple once you're familiar with the basic rules of organizing your wardrobe to suit your personal style, at home and at work. Having a coordinated wardrobe means that your clothes will be more versatile and that you will get a better return on your clothing investment. If t-shirts and jeans are not your idea of casual wear, then maybe a pair of chinos and a casual shirt might be. Not everyone has to wear a suit to work and there is now a business casual style that makes dressing for the office more flexible and comfortable. Whatever your needs, invest in clothes wisely – you'll want to spend more on suits if this is what you wear to work, whereas if you wear a suit only a couple of times a year, think twice about what to spend.

Your wardrobe will contain clothes for every occasion – in varying quantities depending on your job and lifestyle.

The well-dressed man

To transform yourself into the well-dressed man you don't necessarily have to spend a lot of money on clothes or slavishly follow fashion. You simply need to choose clothes that complement your colouring, suit your build, match your personality and are appropriate for whatever occasion you are attending.

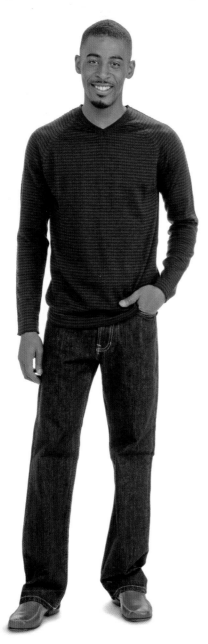

Colour

Since men don't tend to wear make-up they don't have the advantage that women do of being able to make their complexion look flawless. It is therefore important that the colour you wear near your face complements your natural skin tone.

Often, by making subtle changes to the colour of your shirt, not only will you look younger, healthier and fitter, but your '5 o'clock shadow' will disappear, too, and your eyes will sparkle.

By understanding your dominant colouring and how colours work together (see Chapter 2), you will be able to assemble a coordinated wardrobe with fewer clothes but more combinations to wear. Everyone can wear every colour but your individual colouring will affect whether you opt for lighter or darker shades, warm or cool undertones and what strength (clear to muted) that colour should be.

Build

Your basic build relates to your body shape (you will be an Inverted triangle, a Rectangle or Rounded), your scale, height and proportions. Which one of these categories you fall into needs to be taken into consideration when choosing your clothes. For some of you, your scale and proportions may prove a challenge when shopping for clothes, whilst for others this won't be the main factor in dictating your choice because most styles fit you well.

Your body shape will determine the cut of the jackets, shirts and trousers you should be wearing (see Chapter 3) and dictate the fabrics and patterns that best suit you.

Style Personality

By completing the simple questionnaire on pages 74–75, you will be able to identify your style personality – be it Creative, Dramatic, Romantic, Classic, Natural or International. Once you have identified this you will learn from Chapter 4 why a certain style of dressing suits you and your lifestyle, whether you are at work or at leisure. Your style personality will often influence your choice of hobbies, be it sport or something more creative; it will even influence your choice of car.

Appropriateness

There is nothing more embarrassing than arriving at a business appointment or social occasion wearing the wrong clothes. Chapter 5 shows you how to look the part, whatever the occasion, without compromising on your colouring, build and style requirements.

Keeping up to date

This does not necessarily mean following fashion, but simply keeping up to date with the requirements imposed on your wardrobe by your changing age and physique, as well as lifestyle (see pages 156–157).

Men's fashions tend to be cyclical and change normally over a period of a decade, but this does not mean that you only need to shop every 10 years, as the progression is gradual. Shopping for clothes should not be a chore. Pages 138–139 give you a plan to take the stress out of shopping, and will help you learn to differentiate between investment and fashion buys, giving you a wardrobe that works for you with little effort and time.

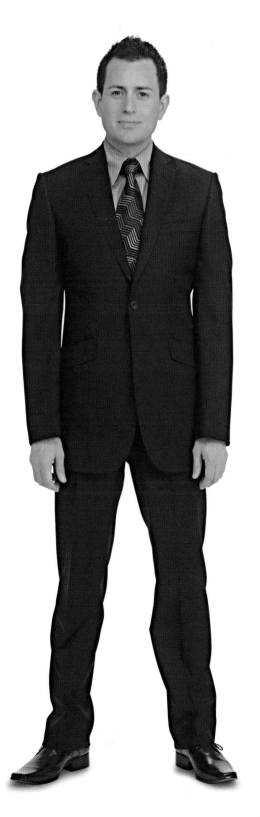

It could be you...

Be inspired by these 'before and after' make-overs. Observe how, by making subtle changes to colour combinations and clothing styles, and some effort in the grooming department, these men have transformed themselves. You, too, can make the most of yourself by taking the advice offered throughout the following chapters.

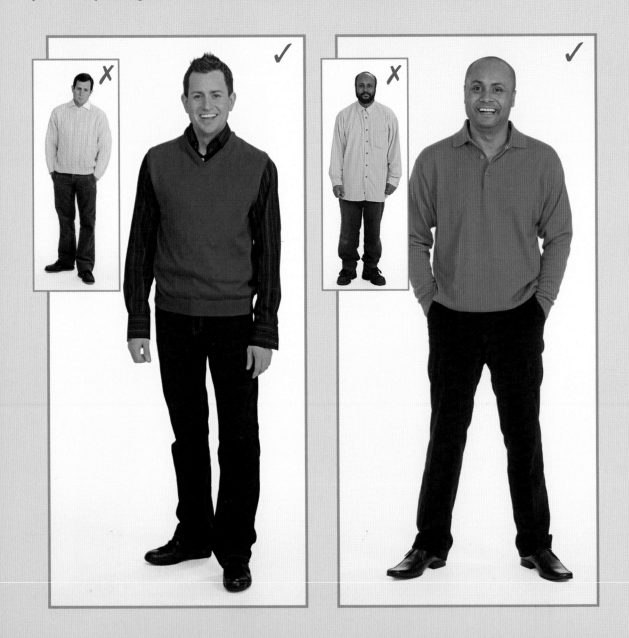

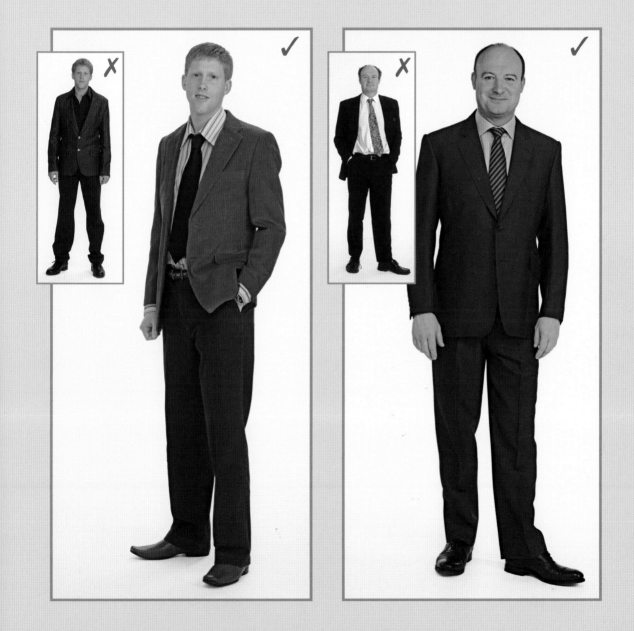

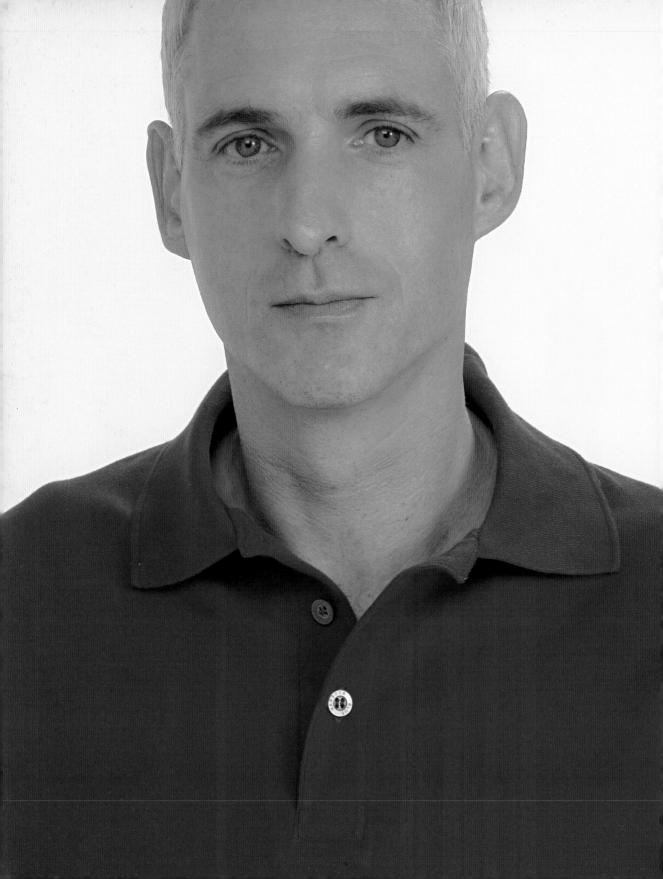

2

how colour
can work
for you

Knowing your colours

Everybody may be described as having one overall dominant colouring characteristic (see pages 20–21). Working out which one best describes you means you can decide which colours are ideal for your wardrobe. In this chapter you will learn how to combine colours and balance them with your own dominant colouring.

Why do you need to know?

When wearing a colour near your face the light reflects upwards, either enhancing your look or casting shadows and making you look tired, unhealthy and older. Wearing the right colour will lighten your complexion, brighten your eyes and give you a healthier appearance. If you don't believe this just try it for yourself. Stand in front of a mirror and observe the miraculous change in your appearance when you exchange a pure white shirt for a cream one, or any icy pink shirt for a peach one.

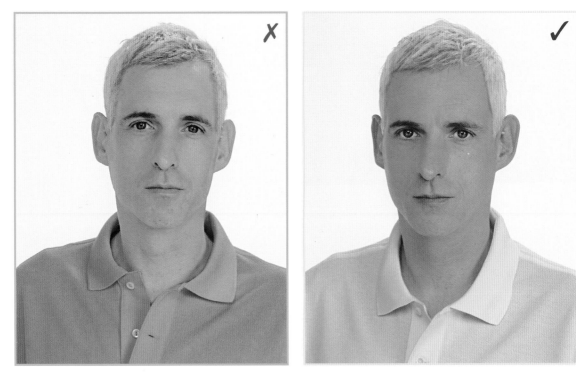

The warm undertone of this peach shirt reflects an unflattering yellow tone on to the skin.

The cool blue-based colour of this shirt makes the complexion appear fresher and eyes brighter.

There are thousands of shades of colour available and some will suit you better than others. Being aware of the variations of shades and tones will help when discovering what suits you best. Blue, for example, can be a pale sky blue or a deep denim blue. Pinks can vary from a pale shell pink to a rich salmon. For many men blue is blue and pink is pink! One of the reasons for this is that colour blindness is more common in men than women, so the subtleties of the variations of shades may not be as obvious to men as they are to women. Indeed, colour blindness seems to occur in eight to 12 per cent of men while only 0.5 per cent of women are afflicted. This is why so many men benefit from having a colour analysis because the guesswork as to which colours to wear is taken away.

Once you know which colours suit you best, shopping for clothes becomes easier. And, when it comes to your casual wardrobe, you will find that you can mix and match all your sweaters, shirts and trousers effortlessly, giving you a greater selection for putting outfits together. Dressing for work will be more enjoyable, too. By cleverly combining shirts and ties with a couple of staple suits, you could have a different look for every day of the week.

Another bonus of knowing your colours is that if anybody else buys your clothes for you, you can tell them exactly what colour suits you.

Understanding your colour type, and taking the time to consider your overall look, will improve your appearance in more ways than one. You may soon have a new approach to your grooming and fitness routines that make for a happier, healthier you, too.

Wearing the right colour near your face reflects light upwards, making you look bright-eyed and healthy.

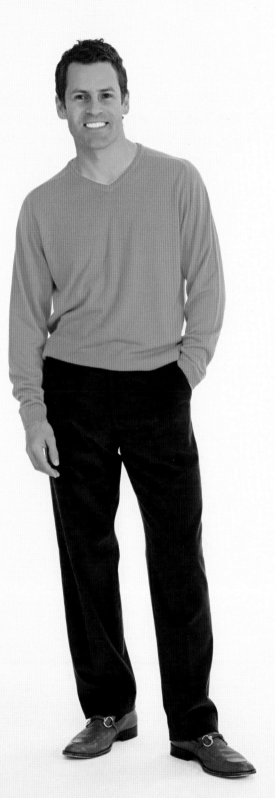

The science of colour

In the 1920s, the Bauhaus artist Johannes Itten revealed in his book, *The Art of Colour*, strong relationships between the way students looked, their personalities and the colours they liked to work with. This concept was further developed at the Los Angeles Fashion Academy, founded in 1972. Ex-student Carole Jackson made the concept popular in her 1980s bestseller *Colour Me Beautiful* and founded the company of the same name.

Since then the organization has developed and fine-tuned the system to make it work not only for women but also for men. In 1984 Carole Jackson wrote *Color For Men*, and in 1993 Mary Spillane's *Presenting Yourself for Men*, was published.

In 2006 *Colour Me Confident* brought to women an updated version of the colour analysis process, using the Munsell system of colour recognition rather than the seasonal concept that **colour me beautiful** had used for the past 25 years.

The Munsell system

The Munsell system is the most widely accepted system of colour measurement in the world. It is used by the British Standards Institution and the US National Bureau of Standards. Its uses are innumerable: the building, printing, hair colouring and automotive industries, for example, utilize it widely. Now, people's colouring (see pages 20–21) can also be described using the Munsell theories.

So, what is Munsell? In 1903, the artist Albert Munsell invented a system of colour identification based on the three responses of the human eye. In 1905 Munsell's 'System of Color Notation' became universally recognized as the language of colours. Colours were identified with three characteristics: hue (undertone), value (depth) and chroma (clarity).

Hue

Hue defines a colour's undertone, which may be warm (yellow-based) or cool (blue-based). Colours such as red, pink or green can be described as having either a warm (yellow) or a cool (blue) undertone. You might

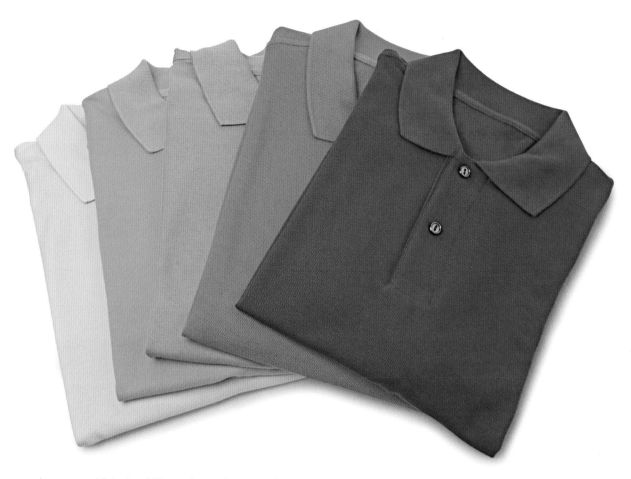

have a cool 'blue' red (like a plum-coloured red), for example, or a warm 'yellow' red (like a tomato red). Use these undertones to your advantage to enhance your natural colouring's tendency to warm or cool.

These polo shirts demonstrate how the same colour can be light, cool, wam, clear or deep.

Value

The value of a colour refers to its depth, giving a measure of its lightness or darkness. Munsell used a scale of 0 to 10 with black being 0 and white being 10, and all the shades of grey in between. This grading of light and dark can be used to measure the depth of all other colours, too. In the home decorating industry, for example, these numbers are used to determine the depth of colour of paint.

Chroma

Chroma indicates the purity, or clarity, of a colour. Some colours are bright and vibrant and reflect the light, while others are muted and seem to absorb the light. The type of fabric will also determine whether light is absorbed or reflected, for example a silk tie reflects light, while a woollen one seems to absorb it.

What's your colouring?

The human eye is always drawn to harmony and balance when looking at the world around us. Just as African animals in the savannah and polar bears in the Arctic are in harmony with their respective environments, so you want to achieve harmony and balance between your physical look and the clothes you wear.

Determining your colouring

Finding your dominant colouring characteristic involves understanding the relationship between your hair, eye and skin tone colouring. The majority of men fall into one of six types – Light, Deep, Warm, Cool, Clear or Muted (see pages 22–45). Unlike women, you don't have the benefit of make-up and hair colouring to define your look. If you find that you fall between two categories, you may need to

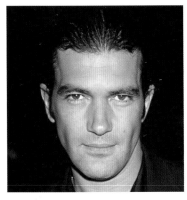

Light

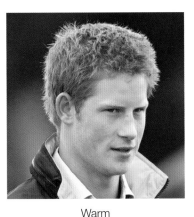

Warm

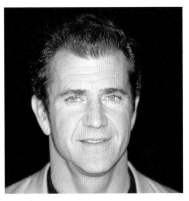

Clear

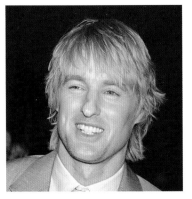

Deep

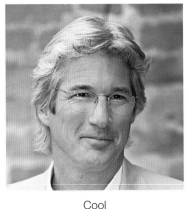

Cool

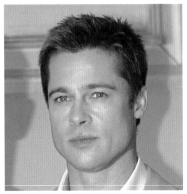

Muted

consider your career and lifestyle. Look at the two palettes and see which one is more appropriate for you; you will also need to refer to the section on colour psychology (see pages 46–47) to help you decide. For example, if you are not sure whether you are Light or Muted, and you are an accountant, you may decide that the Muted palette is a more appropriate one for you.

The picture gallery

The easiest way to decide on your overall dominant colouring characteristic is to go through a process of elimination. Look at the examples opposite and on the following pages and see whose colouring you think you match.

As time goes by…

You might well find that as you get older, your dominant colouring changes. For example, you may have been Deep with a full head of hair, but if your hair thins it is possible you will become Muted as your look will have lightened. Likewise, if you had red hair and it thins, your dominant colouring characteristic may change from Warm to Light.

Most men do not take the route of tinting their hair when the natural highlights begin to show. But be aware that you may need to start to wear some cooler shades near your face.

George Clooney's colouring has changed from deep to cool as he has matured.

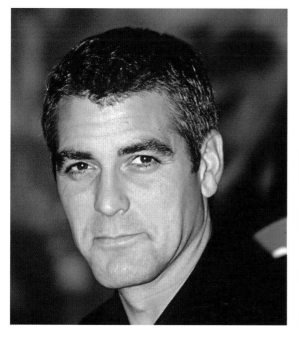
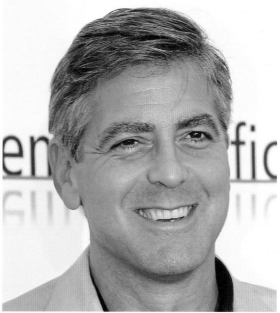

the light man

Your look is pale and youthful. Your skin may be particularly sensitive to chemicals and the sun. Your beard is light. You should always wear a light colour near your face. You need to think carefully about your business look if working in a formal environment, as dark colours will overpower you.

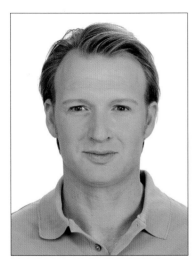

Do you have...

✓ light to medium blond hair – or minimal hair?

✓ blond eyebrows, eye lashes and light beard growth?

✓ pale and delicate skin which can be sensitive ?

✓ pale blue, grey or green eyes?

Wearing colour

Make sure that your overall look is light. When wearing a suit avoid very dark colours and go for medium greys and lighter navies. Keep to the lighter shades in your palette for your shirt and tie combinations.

For casual wear, wear any colours from your palette but use the darker ones for trousers and jackets. When choosing a winter coat, think of pewter or taupe as an alternative to navy or black.

Be careful

Never wear two dark colours together. When wearing a darker colour from your palette always combine it with a lighter shade near your face.

If and when you need a formal business wardrobe, don't choose suits that are too dark.

If you have freckles, choose a shirt with a warm undertone like a light peach, rather than an icy pink.

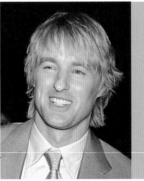

Famous light men

Owen Wilson (pictured)
Sting
Chris Patten
Prince Albert of Monaco
Freddie Flintoff
Vladimir Putin

the colour palette:

neutral colours

light navy

medium charcoal

medium grey

light grey

light denim

pewter

rose brown

cocoa

taupe

stone

sage

petrol

formal shirt colours

soft white

ivory

cream

light apricot

pastel pink

mint

other colours

cornflower

light periwinkle

violet

sky blue

geranium

blush pink

light teal

turquoise

light aqua

peacock

apple green

primrose

the **light** wardrobe: smart

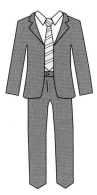

suit: medium grey
shirt: ivory
tie: primrose + ivory

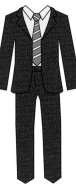

suit: light navy
shirt: mint
tie: turquoise + mint

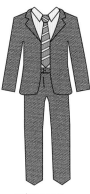

suit: pewter
shirt: light apricot
tie: blush pink
+ light apricot

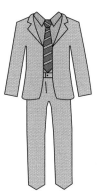

suit: stone
shirt: sky blue
tie: cornflower
+ sky blue

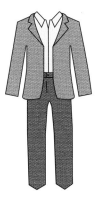

jacket: taupe
shirt: cream
trousers: rose brown

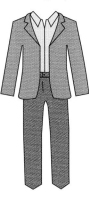

jacket: sage
shirt: pastel pink
trousers: pewter

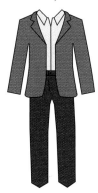

jacket: petrol
shirt: mint
trousers: light navy

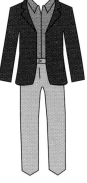

jacket: light navy
shirt: light periwinkle
trousers: stone

Also...

When choosing
shoes, a briefcase,
bag or even a
watchstrap avoid
very dark colours
which will stand
out against the
lighter tones of
your wardrobe.

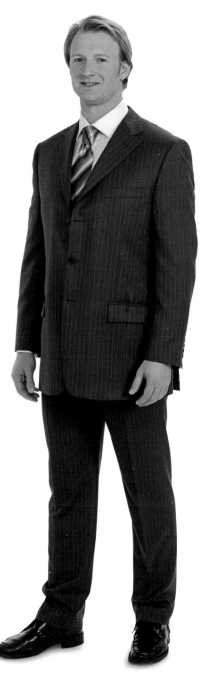

If you wear a dark suit, it's important to
wear light colours near your face.

the **light** wardrobe: casual

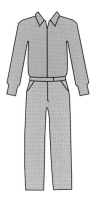

shirt: apple green
chinos: stone

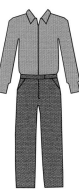

shirt: blush pink
chinos: rose brown

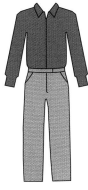

shirt: violet
chinos: sage

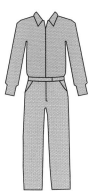

shirt: light aqua
chinos: light grey

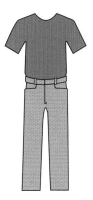

t-shirt: light teal
jeans: sky blue

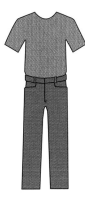

t-shirt: light periwinkle
jeans: cornflower

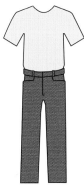

t-shirt: primrose
jeans: petrol

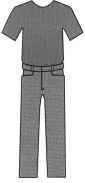

t-shirt: geranium
jeans: medium grey

Also...

When choosing a belt, always ensure the colour is the same as your shoes or tones with your trousers.

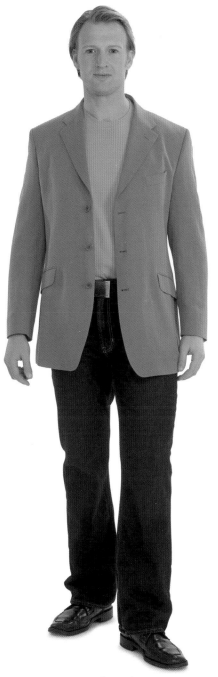

Dark casual trousers are fine as long as your top half is light.

the deep man

Your look is strong and definite. The colours you wear always need to have some strength, or be contrasting. You look good in dark colours worn on their own or dark and light colours worn together, but you should avoid wearing a pale colour on its own near your face.

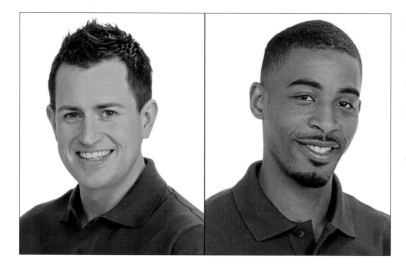

Do you have...

✓ dark brown to black hair?

✓ dark facial hair?

✓ skin ranging from pale to olive through to the darkest brown?

✓ dark eyes?

Wearing colour

Because of your strong look you need to wear strong deep colours. Wearing one dark colour, such as charcoal, from head to toe will look great on you.

When wearing a light coloured shirt, complement it with a dark tie, jacket or sweater to balance your colouring. Your challenge comes in the summer when you are tempted to wear lighter colours. Keep taupe and stone as the colours for your trousers and use a stronger colour near your face.

For your casual wardrobe, if you're wearing just one colour, choose dark or bright shades from your palette and never wear pale colours on their own.

Be careful

The challenge with dark colours is that they get just as dirty as light ones. Be wary of dandruff, hair and dust – there are no shortcuts on the laundry bills for you!

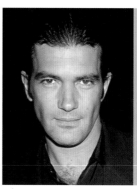

Famous deep men

Antonio Banderas (pictured)
Ben Stiller
Tiger Woods
Ben Affleck
David Schwimmer
Pete Sampras

the colour palette:

neutral colours

black	charcoal	black brown	chocolate	pewter	taupe
dark navy	dark denim	aubergine	pine	teal	stone

formal shirt colours

soft white	ivory	light peach	powder pink	mint	icy violet

other colours

cornflower	true blue	burgundy	bittersweet	scarlet	blush pink
royal purple	forest	emerald	turquoise	fern	lime

the **deep** wardrobe: smart

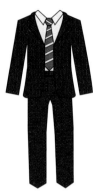

suit: dark navy
shirt: mint
tie: teal + mint

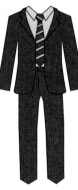

suit: charcoal
shirt: icy violet
tie: burgundy + icy violet

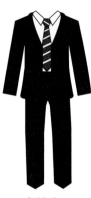

suit: black
shirt: ivory
tie: charcoal + ivory

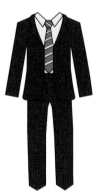

suit: black brown
shirt: light peach
tie: bittersweet
+ light peach

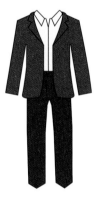

jacket: pine
shirt: soft white
trousers: black brown

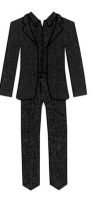

jacket: burgundy
shirt: aubergine
trousers: charcoal

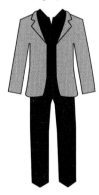

jacket: taupe
shirt: black
trousers: black

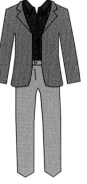

jacket: pewter
shirt: chocolate
trousers: taupe

Also...

When wearing dark trousers make sure your footwear is dark, too. When wearing lighter trousers your footwear needs to be in a complementary shade to the trousers (and socks).

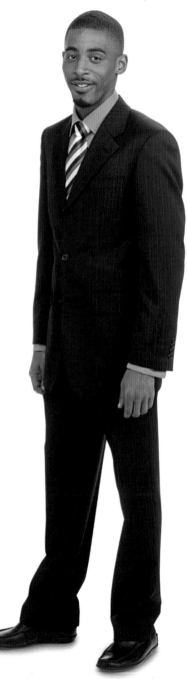

A dark suit should be teamed with dark accessories, such as black shoes.

the **deep** wardrobe: casual

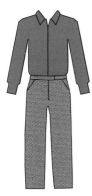

shirt: bittersweet
chinos: pewter

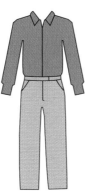

shirt: turquoise
chinos: stone

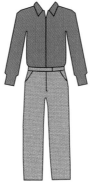

shirt: fern
chinos: taupe

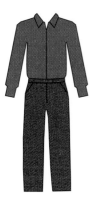

shirt: true blue
chinos: charcoal

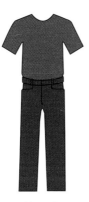

t-shirt: teal
jeans: burgundy

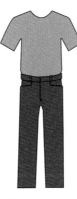

t-shirt: lime
jeans: forest green

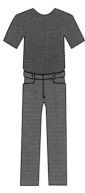

t-shirt: royal purple
jeans: cornflower

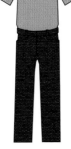

t-shirt: blush pink
jeans: dark navy

Also...
Colour can be
introduced to
a dark outfit
by adding
a colourful bag
or jacket.

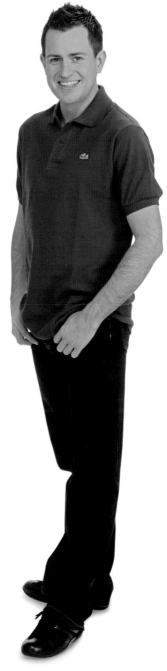

Wearing clothes of a dark colour from head
to toe looks very striking on a Deep man.

the warm man

Your overall appearance has a golden look about it. The colours you wear need to have a warm undertone to them, which means they are yellow-based. You must remember that when you wear navies and greys near your face, you need to warm them up by combining them with warmer colours, such as yellows, peaches and greens.

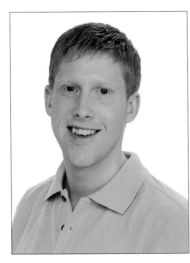

Do you have...

✓ ginger blonde, auburn or red-toned hair?

✓ a beard that grows gingery and perhaps ginger eyebrows?

✓ pale skin with freckles?

✓ blue, green or brown eyes, perhaps with yellow flecks in them?

Wearing colour

As a Warm man, all the colours in your palette are yellow-based. You also have a selection of both Muted and Clear colours to choose from. When wearing colours near your face you can opt for tone on tone, or contrasting shades will also work well.

You may feel more comfortable in a darker tonal look. Don't be afraid to introduce some ambers and reds into your casual wardrobe.

If you have light blue or green eyes, keep to the lighter side of your palette near your face. If you have brown or dark green eyes, you will look better in slightly darker shades near your face.

Be careful

When choosing your pinks and reds make sure that they are yellow-based like bittersweet or terracotta and other tonal reds.

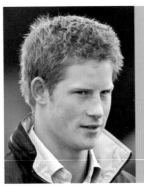

Famous warm men

Prince Harry (pictured)
Damian Lewis
Mick Hucknall
Gene Wilder
Charles Dance

the colour palette:

neutral colours

dark navy	charcoal	pewter	chocolate	bronze	oatmeal
olive	moss	sage	grey green	stone	medium denim

formal shirt colours

soft white	cream	light peach	buttermilk	mint	primrose

other colours

apricot	daffodil	amber	tangerine	terracotta	bittersweet
teal	lime	turquoise	aqua	light periwinkle	purple

the **warm** wardrobe: smart

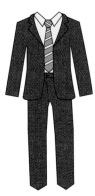

suit: charcoal
shirt: primrose
tie: aqua + primrose

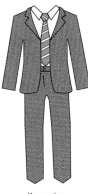

suit: dark navy
shirt: light peach
tie: terracotta + light peach

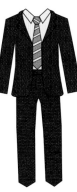

suit: pewter
shirt: buttermilk
tie: lime + buttermilk

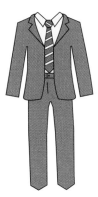

suit: grey green
shirt: cream
tie: moss + cream

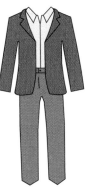

jacket: bronze
shirt: mint
trousers: grey green

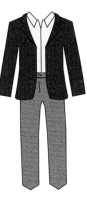

jacket: chocolate
shirt: cream
trousers: pewter

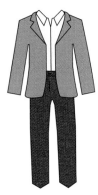

jacket: oatmeal
shirt: soft white
trousers: charcoal

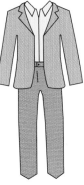

jacket: stone
shirt: primrose
trousers: sage

Also...

If you wear a navy or charcoal suit your shoes need to be black. If you wear navy or charcoal casual trousers, however, your shoes can be brown. Don't forget that the colour of your belt should match that of your shoes.

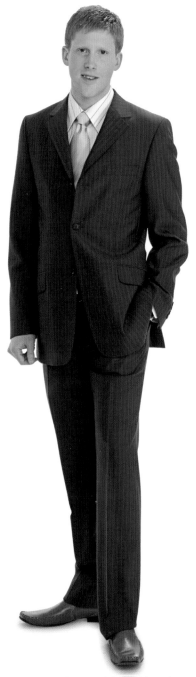

A chocolate brown suit is lifted by using a lime tie and tan coloured shoes.

the **warm** wardrobe: casual

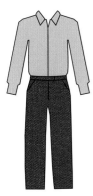

shirt: apricot
chinos: olive

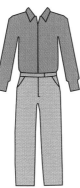

shirt: aqua
chinos: stone

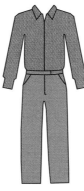

shirt: light periwinkle
chinos: oatmeal

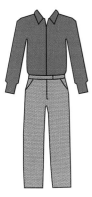

shirt: bittersweet
chinos: sage

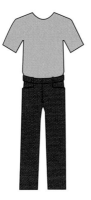

t-shirt: amber
jeans: light navy

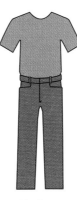

t-shirt: lime
jeans: moss

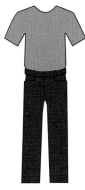

t-shirt: terracotta
jeans: chocolate

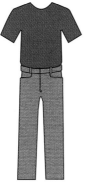

t-shirt: purple
jeans: light periwinkle

Also…

The accessories for your casual wardrobe are best kept to browns and tans. Gold is the ideal choice for frames and watch straps.

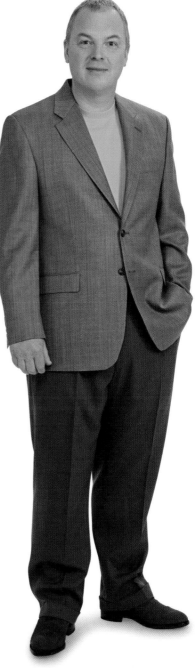

The warm tones of amber and oatmeal are complemented by brown suede shoes.

the cool man

There are more Cool men than women because as men age, they don't usually hide their greying temples. You look good in all shades of grey, navy and blue; pinks and lilacs are also excellent for you. All your colours need to have a cool (blue) undertone – avoid anything yellow-based. This palette works particularly well in a business environment.

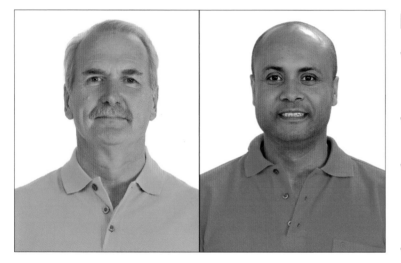

Do you have...

✓ salt and pepper, grey or white hair, or black hair without a hint of red in it?

✓ facial hair that is either black with flecks of grey, or white?

✓ rosy or pink tones to the skin if you're Caucasian and a bluish/greyish undertone to the skin if you are black?

✓ blue, grey or cool brown eyes?

Wearing colour

As a Cool man, all the colours in your palette are blue-based. You also need to have a selection of both Muted and Clear shades and to think about putting your colours together with some contrast.

If you have pale blue eyes and white hair, avoid wearing black near your face. For those of you with dark skin and dark eyes or steely grey hair, you will look better wearing the darker shades of your palette or contrasting colours. If you have light eyes and white hair, choose the pastel colours from your palette.

Cream shirts are not very flattering for your skin tone, so choose icy shades from your palette instead.

Be careful

When choosing your greens make sure they are blue-based (like pine green) rather than yellow-based (like olive green).

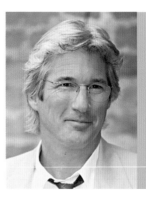

Famous cool men

Richard Gere (pictured)
Sean Connery
Sir Bob Geldof
Junichiro Koizumi
Nelson Mandela
Martin Sheen

the colour palette:

neutral colours

black	charcoal	medium grey	light grey	pewter	taupe

dark navy	sapphire	dark denim	pine	spruce	teal

formal shirt colours

soft white	icy pink	icy grey	icy violet	icy blue	icy green

other colours

duck egg	light aqua	bluebell	sky blue	powder pink	rose pink

sea green	light teal	light periwinkle	purple	cassis	blue red

the **cool** wardrobe: smart

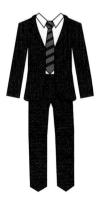

suit: dark navy
shirt: soft white
tie: blue red + navy

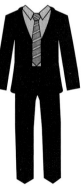

suit: black
shirt: light grey
tie: light periwinkle
+ light grey

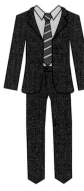

suit: charcoal
shirt: icy violet
tie: purple
+ icy violet

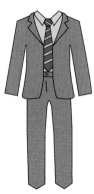

suit: medium grey
shirt: powder pink
tie: cassis
+ powder pink

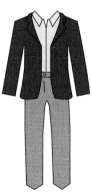

jacket: sapphire
shirt: bluebell
trousers: charcoal

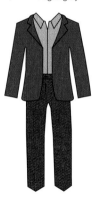

jacket: pine
shirt: icy green
trousers: taupe

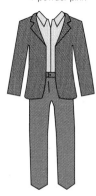

jacket: pewter
shirt: icy grey
trousers: medium grey

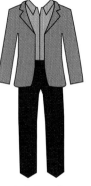

jacket: medium grey
shirt: sky blue
trousers: dark navy

Also...
For spectacles,
watch straps and
wedding rings,
choose from the
silver, steel and
titanium range.

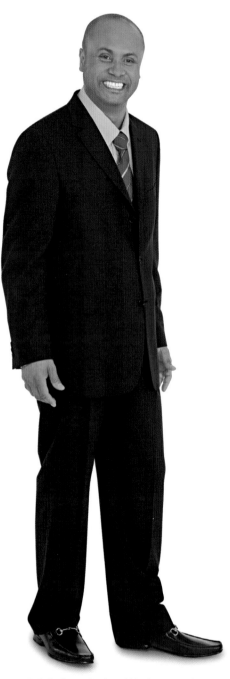

A dark charcoal suit and black accessories
are perfectly teamed with a pink shirt.

the **cool** wardrobe: casual

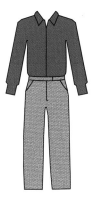

shirt: cassis
chinos: taupe

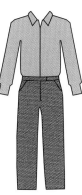

shirt: duck egg
chinos: pewter

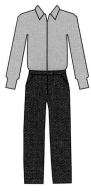

shirt: rose pink
chinos: charcoal

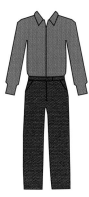

shirt: light teal
chinos: spruce

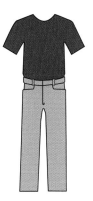

t-shirt: sapphire
jeans: sea green

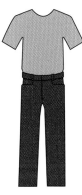

t-shirt: light aqua
jeans: pine

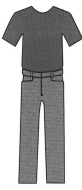

t-shirt: blue red
jeans: medium grey

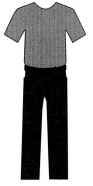

t-shirt: light periwinkle
jeans: black

Also...

Take care with the colour of your shoes with your casual wardrobe. Avoid tan browns and select red browns, like oxblood, instead.

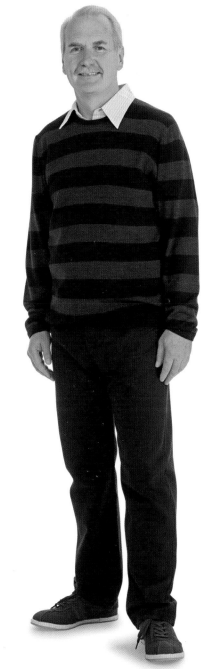

Navy blue, denim tones or grey are a great alternative to black for your casual look.

the clear man

You have one of the most dramatic looks, often with dark hair, bright eyes and light or dark skin. With such a striking appearance you look great in contrasting colours and can mix light and dark colours with confidence. The sludgy colours in your palette, like taupe and pewter, should be mixed with bright colours for best effect.

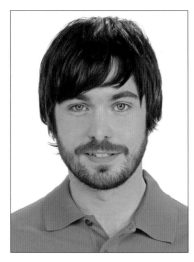

Do you have...

✓ dark hair?

✓ dark eyebrows and lashes?

✓ pale skin, possibly with a few freckles, or darker skin with a clear complexion?

✓ bright blue, green, topaz or clear brown eyes?

Wearing colour

Wear colours that are contrasting: the darker the jacket and trousers, the brighter or lighter the shirt should be. Ties always need to contrast with and complement the colour of your shirt.

When choosing a shirt or sweater, opt for one of the brighter shades, or even pure white, and wear it with dark trousers.

If wearing just one colour, make sure it is bright and clear. If wearing pewter, charcoal, chocolate or stone near your face they will need to be balanced with contrasting shades, such as a Chinese blue sweater or a light teal jacket.

Be careful

If your skin has a warm look, go for shirt colours like light apricot and peach; if you have a cooler skin tone, you will look better in the icy colours of your palette.

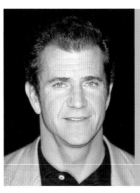

Famous clear men

Mel Gibson (pictured)
Tom Cruise
Pierce Brosnan
Robbie Williams
Hugh Grant
Eddie Murphy
Jeremy Irons

the colour palette:

neutral colours

black	charcoal	medium grey	light grey	dark navy	royal blue
black brown	chocolate	pewter	stone	dark denim	evergreen

formal shirt colours

soft white	ivory	light peach	mint	icy violet	sky blue

other colours

true blue	Chinese blue	cornflower	bright periwinkle	purple	blush pink
light teal	emerald turquoise	apple green	duck egg	light aqua	scarlet

the **clear** wardrobe: smart

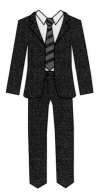

suit: charcoal
shirt: light peach
tie: scarlet + charcoal

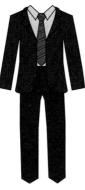

suit: dark navy
shirt: icy violet
tie: bright periwinkle + purple

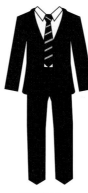

suit: black
shirt: soft white
tie: black + light grey

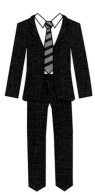

suit: black brown
shirt: ivory
tie: emerald turquoise + black brown

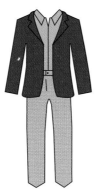

jacket: royal blue
shirt: duck egg
trousers: light grey

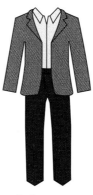

jacket: pewter
shirt: mint
trousers: black brown

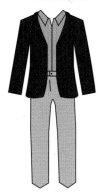

jacket: dark navy
shirt: sky blue
trousers: stone

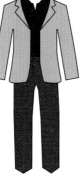

jacket: light grey
shirt: black
trousers: charcoal

Also...

If you have a few freckles and maybe some red in your hair, avoid the icy colours from your palette for shirts; if you have a cooler and rosier complexion, avoid wearing lemon yellow near your face.

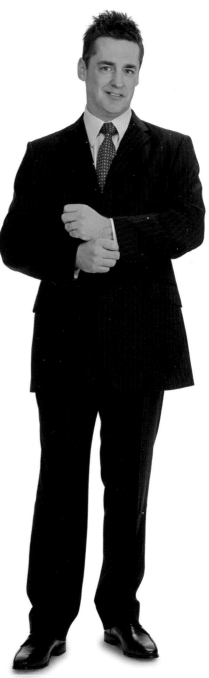

Pick out a contrasting tone in a pinstripe suit for a coordinated effect.

the **clear** wardrobe: casual

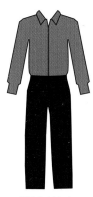

shirt: light teal
chinos: black

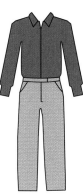

shirt: Chinese blue
chinos: stone

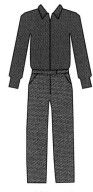

shirt: purple
chinos: pewter

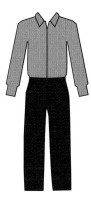

shirt: blush pink
chinos: dark navy

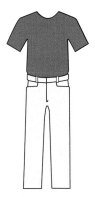

t-shirt: scarlet
jeans: ivory

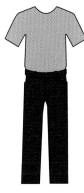

t-shirt: light aqua
jeans: dark navy

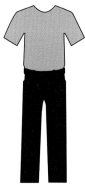

t-shirt: apple green
jeans: black

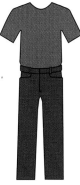

t-shirt: cornflower
jeans: royal blue

Also...

Brighten up your casual look with accessories in bright colours. Try a sports bag in vibrant red, green or blue.

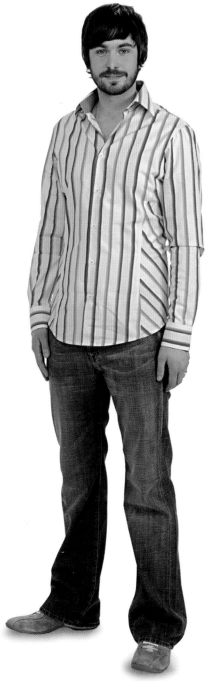

Use your colour palette to choose casual shirts with complementary stripes.

the muted man

Your overall look is not well defined and you may have found a little of you in some of the other dominants. The key to your look is to avoid strong bright colours, particularly when worn in contrast. To balance with your medium-depth colouring you will look better in tonal hues. Soft white or ivory is a good choice for business shirts.

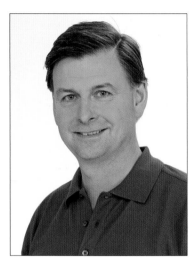

Do you have...

✓ dark blond to mid-brown hair?

✓ dark blond to dark brown eyebrows and lashes?

✓ light to olive skin?

✓ blended tones of blue, green, grey or brown eyes?

Wearing colour

Your colours are best when they are of medium depth. When choosing shirt and tie combinations, the colours need to be tonal, either one shade lighter or one shade darker. The stark, pure white shirt is not a good look for you.

Remember that the texture of the fabrics of your shirts, jackets, ties and tops will soften the colours. Fabrics that are loosely woven or knitted work well. Patterns in ties and shirts need to look blended with no high contrast.

As natural highlights start to show at the temples, consider colours from the cool palette.

Be careful

For your business look avoid very dark navies together with a white shirt and a bright tie; your navy needs to be an obvious navy rather than a black navy.

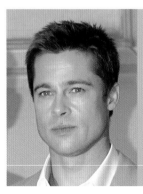

Famous muted men

Brad Pitt (pictured)
Jamie Oliver
David Beckham
Jamie Cullum
Bill Gates
Jude Law
Hugh Laurie

the colour palette:

neutral colours

light navy	charcoal	charcoal blue	medium denim	pewter	grey green

chocolate	rose brown	cocoa	taupe	stone	natural beige

formal shirt colours

soft white	ivory	light peach	shell	mint	sky blue

other colours

sage	verbena	jade	turquoise	teal	emerald turquoise

sapphire	light periwinkle	bluebell	soft violet	purple	claret

the **muted** wardrobe: smart

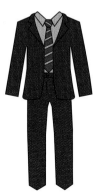

suit: light navy
shirt: sky blue
tie: sapphire + sky blue

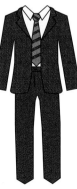

suit: charcoal
shirt: soft white
tie: jade + charcoal

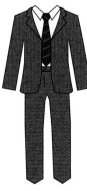

suit: blue charcoal
shirt: ivory
tie: navy + blue charcoal

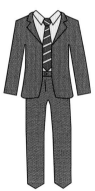

suit: rose brown
shirt: shell
tie: claret + shell

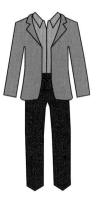

jacket: cocoa
shirt: sage
trousers: chocolate

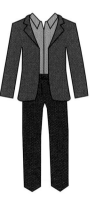

jacket: teal
shirt: verbena
trousers: light navy

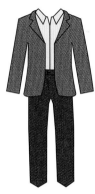

jacket: pewter
shirt: light peach
trousers: charcoal

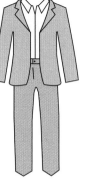

jacket: natural beige
shirt: ivory
trousers: stone

Also...
Black accessories, such as shoes or a briefcase, will work with your charcoals and navies.

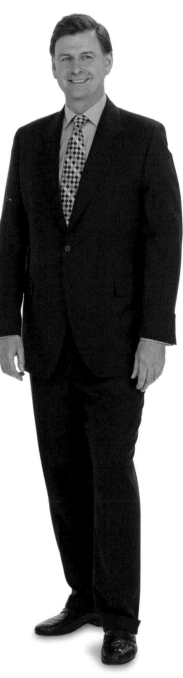

A woven silk tie will soften the effect of a dark-coloured suit.

the **muted** wardrobe: casual

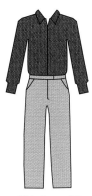

shirt: charcoal blue
chinos: stone

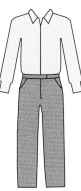

shirt: mint
chinos: taupe

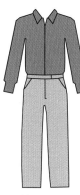

shirt: turquoise
chinos: natural beige

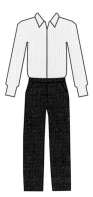

shirt: light peach
chinos: chocolate

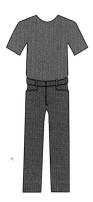

t-shirt: soft violet
jeans: purple

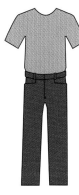

t-shirt: sky blue
jeans: sapphire

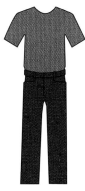

t-shirt: rose brown
jeans: chocolate

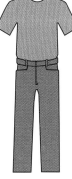

t-shirt: sage
jeans: grey green

Also...

Because your look is tonal, avoid black accessories for casual wear. Opt for brown or beige suede shoes instead of black leather.

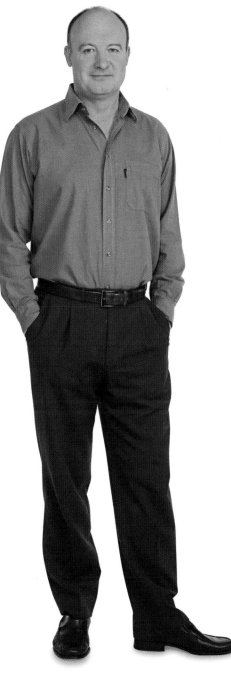

Muted, earthy tones are ideally suited to softer fabrics for casual wear.

Colour psychology

Men are sometimes wary of using colour in their wardrobe, so the only items of colour tend to be their ties. However, a basic understanding of simple colour psychology may give you the confidence to buy the pink shirt you have always shied away from. You should also be aware that the colours you wear may have an impact on others.

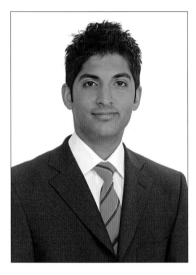

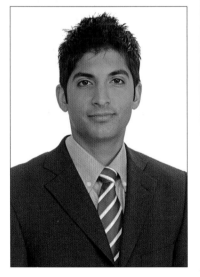

The high contrast in the top picture is authoritative, while the tonal shades in the picture above are approachable.

Black and reds

Black and red are both seen as colours of authority and assertiveness. Either colour worn on its own gives out these signals; wear both colours together and you will appear one powerful man!

If you wear a black shirt, keep it casual, as a formal black shirt may convey the wrong message. Charcoals and medium greys are more approachable than black.

Whether you are choosing a casual shirt or a tie, make sure you get the right red for your colouring, for example raspberry and burgundy are blue-based, tomato and red orange are yellow-based. Wearing a red tie will have an energizing effect on you and those who see it – choose this colour if you want to make sure your point of view gets across.

Browns and beiges

At one time it was considered that no man of standing should wear a brown suit. With globalization and the mixing of cultures, however, brown is now acceptable in many more professions.

Brown gives out a more relaxed, more approachable message than black. In warm climates, all tones of beige are perfectly acceptable for business wear. It is important, however, to wear the right tones. If you are a Deep or Clear, wear your beige jacket with a darker or brighter shirt colour from your palette.

The beige raincoat is a uniform for many men and works perfectly well worn over any other colour.

If greying, avoid yellow tones in your beiges, taupes and camels. Stone and pewter will work better.

Blue is the most popular colour for men to wear, being safe and conservative yet authoritative. Pink exudes confidence and suggests that you are comfortable with your masculinity, yet shows compassion.

Navies and blues

These are the most popular colours for men to wear, being safe and conservative yet authoritative. Blue also communicates trustworthiness, together with peace and order. This is why navy appears in so many uniforms.

Navies and blues are easy and simple to match, for example wear navy with a white or blue shirt.

If you are wearing a blue shirt as part of a formal look, make sure you include some blue in your tie to complement and coordinate with your shirt. Don't forget that turquoises and aquas are blues, too.

Denim is easily combined with any other colour from your wardrobe. Men with a Deep or Clear colouring should choose the darker shades of denim to ensure a balanced overall look.

Greens and yellows

The colour of nature, green is popular with the armed forces and proves perfect for camouflage. It gives out a reassuring message, and certain shades of green have a calming effect, hence green is often chosen by institutions for uniforms and wall colour.

Greens vary from blue-based hues (like pine and teal) to yellow-based ones (like olive and moss). The brighter shades of green are best used either for casual wear or as an accent colour in a tie.

Yellow, from lemon to mustard, is a friendly and approachable colour which, over the past decade, has become increasingly popular and acceptable as a formal shirt colour. Men with grey hair should limit their use of yellow to an accent colour (a spot, a stripe or a check).

Pinks and purples

A man who wears pink exudes confidence and is comfortable with his masculinity, yet shows that he has compassion.

Choose your pink carefully, remembering that it can vary from a warm salmon pink (which is yellow-based) to an icy pink or raspberry (which are blue-based). Pink is a great colour for a casual shirt worn at the weekend, helping you to unwind and relax.

Purple varies from damson to icy violet and communicates creativity and modernity. If you have never worn a colour from the purple family before, try it in a tie or t-shirt and see what compliments you receive.

If you are not comfortable wearing pink, try icy violet, violet or shades of lavender.

As you grey, all shades of pinks and purples will flatter and even out your skin tone.

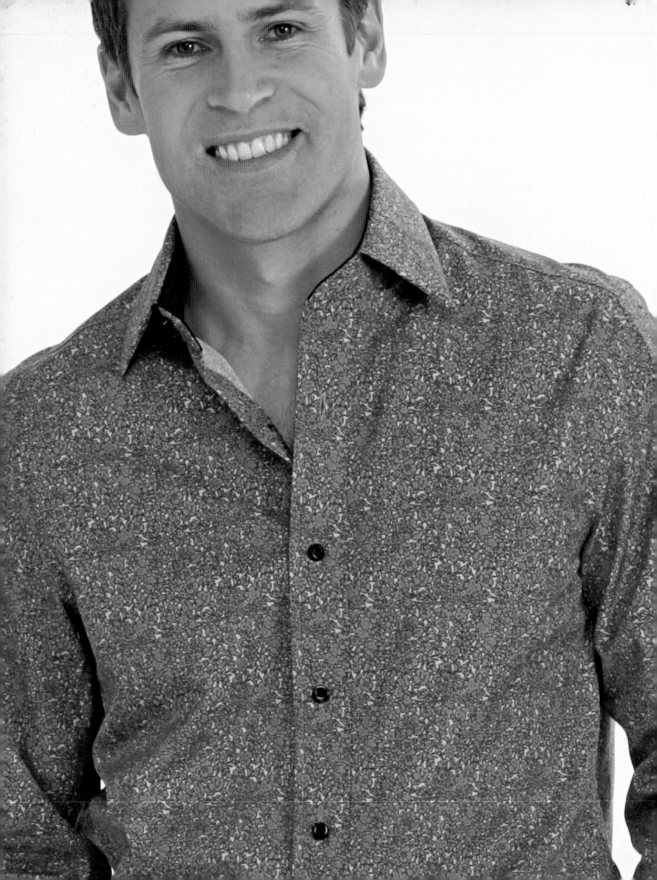

3

dressing for your build

What's your body shape?

Beneath your clothes your body has a certain shape that you need to consider when you are shopping for clothes. This chapter takes you, step by step, through the elements of understanding your body shape, scale and proportions and offers guidelines to being that well-dressed man.

Consider how lucky you are: a man's body is much easier to dress than a woman's as your overall shape is much more streamlined. By identifying your body shape you will know what cut or style of clothes you should wear. This applies to all the items in your wardrobe – from formal suits to your holiday shorts.

To identify your basic body shape, answer the questions next to each illustration, then turn to the relevant section (see pages 52–63) to find the guidelines for clothes that suit your shape.

Did you know?...

Fabric The texture and weight of the fabrics you wear need to be in balance with your build.

Pattern Patterns on sweaters, ties and shirts can affect your overall look so ensure they balance with your scale (see pages 64–65).

Your size Don't assume that your waist measurement will be the same when you are 40, for example, as it was in your 20s, even if the bathroom scales show that you haven't gained weight.

Fit Not all manufacturers' clothing sizes are the same, so, when buying a major item, make sure you try it on first to ensure you have the correct fit (see pages 116–119).

Inverted triangle

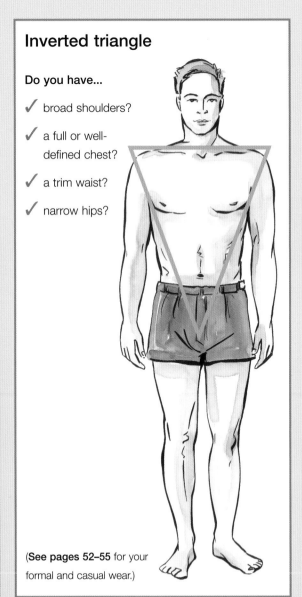

Do you have...

✓ broad shoulders?

✓ a full or well-defined chest?

✓ a trim waist?

✓ narrow hips?

(**See pages 52–55** for your formal and casual wear.)

Before clothes shopping in earnest you need to decide what shape your body is – whether it is triangular, rectangular or rounded. These guidelines will help you to decide which type best describes your shape.

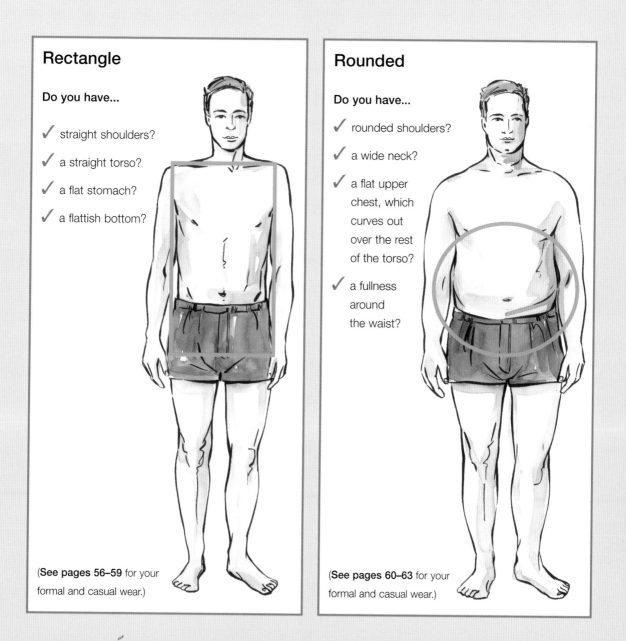

Rectangle

Do you have...

✓ straight shoulders?

✓ a straight torso?

✓ a flat stomach?

✓ a flattish bottom?

(See pages 56–59 for your formal and casual wear.)

Rounded

Do you have...

✓ rounded shoulders?

✓ a wide neck?

✓ a flat upper chest, which curves out over the rest of the torso?

✓ a fullness around the waist?

(See pages 60–63 for your formal and casual wear.)

Inverted triangle – formal wear

Your overall stature is impressive with your broad upper body and narrow hips. Your challenge in getting the correct fit is to avoid obscuring your silhouette, which needs to remain uncluttered. Men, like American sportsman Michael Johnson, know how to dress to show off their physique, keeping the lines of their clothes simple yet striking.

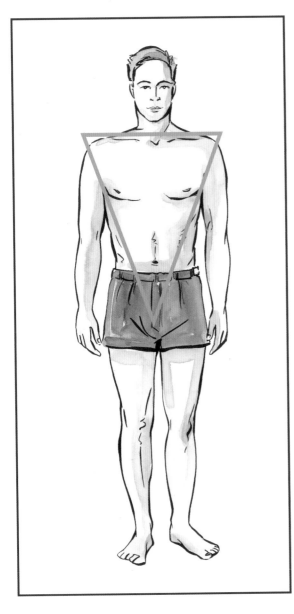

Your key rule

✓ Keep the overall look sharp, simple and uncluttered.

Suits, jackets and trousers

Crisp, clean lines are essential and finely woven fabrics will achieve these.

Your best styles

The overall look of the suit needs to be sharp and crisp. This can be achieved with either tailoring or fabric. Most suit styles look good on you, however the Italian cut will show off your physique best (see pages 104–109).

A double-breasted blazer or sports jacket with wider lapels will suit you.

Front-pleated trousers and/or wider legs will balance your shoulder line.

Your best fabrics

Finely woven plain or patterned (see below) fabrics, such as:
Gabardine
Fine wool worsted
Lightweight twill

Your best patterns

The size of pattern you should wear depends on your scale (see page 64):

Pinstripes
Herringbone
Prince of Wales
Windowpane
Houndstooth

Shirts

A plain crisp cotton shirt and a stiff collar will always work well.

Your best fabrics

Fine cotton
Two-fold poplin

Your best patterns

End to end
Stripes
Checks
Graph checks
Gingham

Ties

Make sure the pattern is angular and the size of pattern suits your scale – see page 64.

Your best fabrics

Plain or woven silk

Your best patterns

Stripes
Geometric patterns
Checks
Dots

You should avoid

✗ Heavy and bulky fabrics, floral patterns and the American-style deconstructed suit (see page 109).

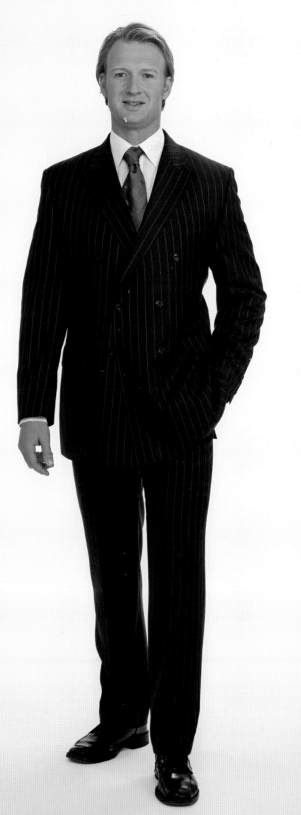

Inverted triangle – casual wear

Just because you are donning your casual clothes it doesn't mean that you should forget about the basic rules of keeping your clothing lines simple and uncluttered. Even when wearing more than one layer, make sure your silhouette remains visible, so avoid bulky clothes, such as chunky knit jumpers.

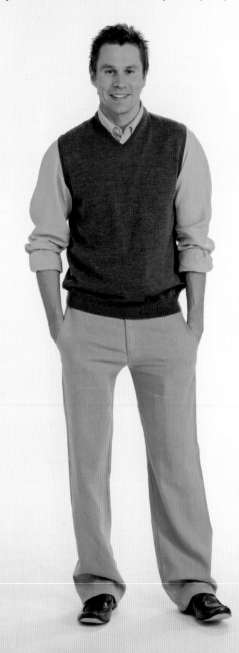

Your key rule

✓ Aim to show off your wide shoulders and slim hips. Go for reasonably close-fitting clothes rather than baggy ones, unless they are tucked in.

Jackets

Choose jackets with some structure and in crisp fabrics that will retain their shape.

Your best styles
Shaped jackets

An inserted sleeve and notch collar will add structure to your jacket.

Your best fabrics
Linen
Denim
Heavy cotton twill
Fine needlecord
Leather
Waxed

Trousers

Pocket details on trousers are good but make sure
they lie flat so that they don't break your silhouette.

Your best styles
Flat-fronted trousers or jeans

Your best fabrics
Denim
Wool
Heavy cotton or wool twill
Fine needlecord

Tops

Your shoulders are one of your best features, so make
sure the shoulder line is visible.

Your best styles
T-shirts
Polo shirts
Roll-necks
V-necks with inserted sleeves

Your best fabrics
Fine to medium knits
Oxford cloth
Cotton twill
Linen

Your best patterns

All stripes and checks are good patterns for you to
wear on shirts or sweaters.

You should avoid

✗ Blouson jackets, baggy shirts and t-shirts,
heavy-knit sweaters, soft and floppy knits and
flowery patterns.

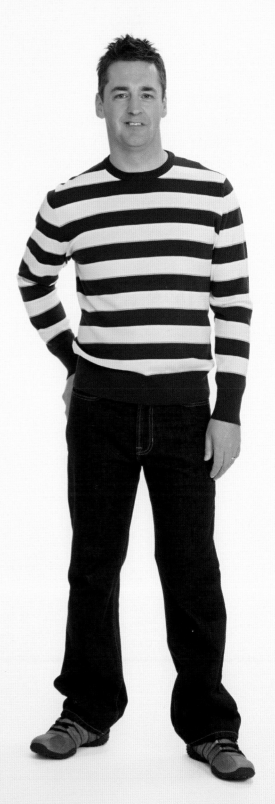

Rectangle – formal wear

You can walk into a store and buy an off-the-peg suit without any problems. However, it is important to ensure that the scale and proportions are right for your height and build. Your choice of fabrics and patterns will also depend on your scale (see pages 64–65). Golfer Tiger Woods, has a rectangular build and wears his clothes with style.

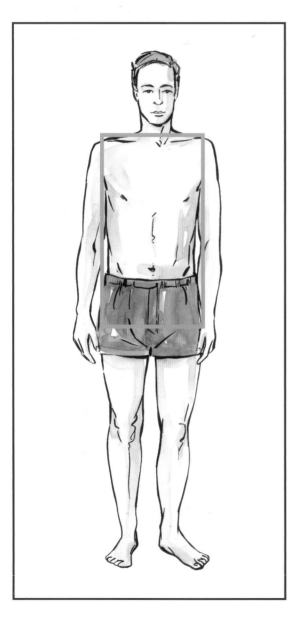

Your key rule

✓ Ensure you get the proper fit for your scale and proportions (see pages 64–67).

Suits, jackets and trousers

Most styles will suit you, just make sure the fit is right for your body shape (see pages 116–119).

Your best styles
The best clothing line for you is lean and slightly shaped around the waist, rather than falling straight down from the armpits.

The British-cut style of suit is best for you (see page 107).

Both single- or double-breasted jackets will suit you well, depending on your height and proportions (see pages 64–67).

Pleated or flat-fronted trousers are good for you, whichever you find the most comfortable.

Your best fabrics
Whether plain or patterned, the best fabrics that will drape well over a rectangular shape are:
Worsted
Twill
Medium-weight flannel
Lightweight tweed

Your best patterns

Medium-weight stripes

Bird's eye

Prince of Wales

Herringbone

Windowpane

Puppy-, Dog- or Houndstooth depending on your scale

Shirts

Wear your city shirts for your more formal look teamed
with a simply patterned tie.

Your best fabrics

Cotton or cotton twill

Two-fold poplin

Your best patterns

Checks or gingham

Stripes or graphic print

Herringbone

Windowpane

Ties

Ensure the colours in your tie pick out at least one
colour from your shirt.

Your best fabrics

Plain or woven silk

Plain or patterned knit

Your best patterns

Foulard

Club

Motifs

Spots

Paisley

You should avoid

✗ Bulky and heavy fabrics, a sloppy shoulder line
and large lapels.

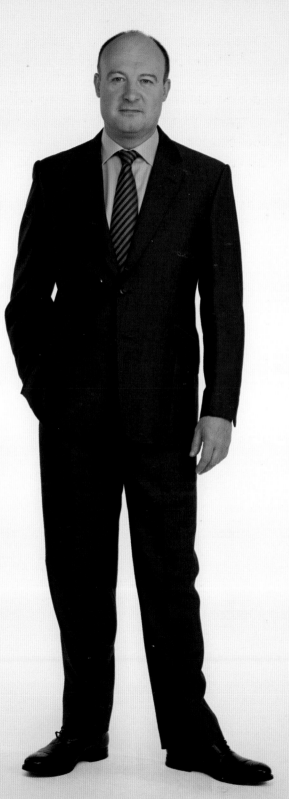

Rectangle – casual wear

As a Rectangle, you have the widest selection of casual styles to choose from when shopping. Your main priority is to ensure that your clothes are appropriate for the occasion and suit your personality. Remember, just because clothes continue to fit you with the passing of time, it doesn't mean that they shouldn't be updated occasionally.

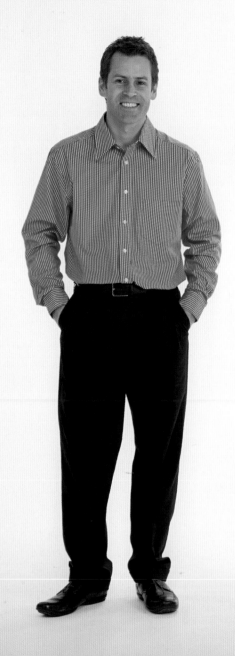

Your key rules

✓ Both fitted and looser-fitting clothes are good for you. You want to feel comfortable in your casual clothes, but don't compromise your look by completely disguising your build.

Jackets

Ensure the jacket does not swamp you around the arms or chest area.

Your best styles
All styles of jackets suit you, from blazers to denim, as long as they fit you properly.

Your best fabrics
Linen
Denim
Cashmere mix
Corduroy
Suede
Leather
Heavy cotton twill
Tweed
Waxed
Fleece

Trousers

You need a selection of casual trousers to allow for various casual looks and different occasions.

Your best styles
All styles of trousers look good on you, providing you follow the rules of proportions (see pages 66–67).

Your best fabrics
Denim
Corduroy
Cotton or wool twill
Moleskin
Flannel
Linen

Tops

Tops do not stop at shirts. Allow for various styles from t-shirts to sleeveless v-necks (see pages 141–142).

Your best styles
Leaving your top untucked may not be your best look (see 'Your Proportions', pages 66–67).

Your best fabrics
Fine to medium cotton or wool knits
Brushed cotton
Linen
Silk
Chambray
Cheesecloth

Your best patterns

Any pattern is good for you as long as it is appropriate for your scale (see page 64).

You should avoid

✗ Belted cardigans and overlayering.

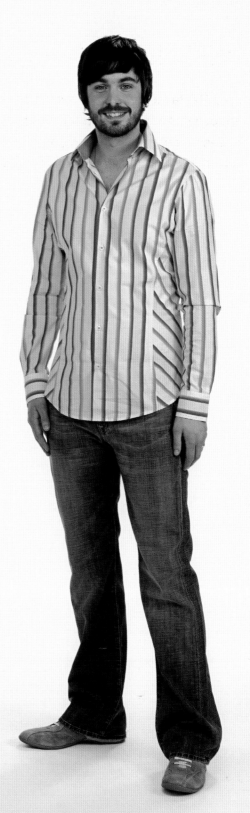

Rounded – formal wear

You have a contoured and cuddly physique. Your shape may be predetermined by your genes, or the force of gravity may have taken its toll. Fabric is your main consideration when choosing clothes, as your silhouette needs to be gently contoured. American actor Danny De Vito achieves this comfortable look while remaining well dressed.

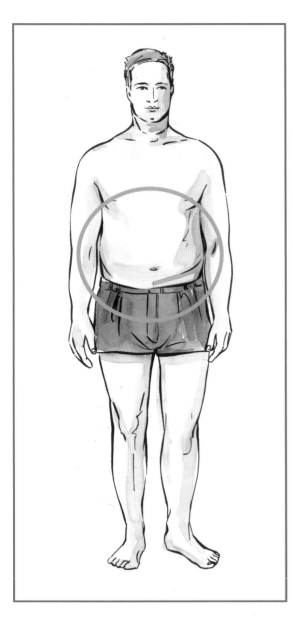

Your key rule

✓ You must think carefully about the fabrics you select when buying your clothes.

Suits, jackets and trousers

American cut soft styling in relaxed fabrics will suit your body shape best.

Your best styles

Generally, softer tailoring is better for you – no hard lines or close-fitting clothes.

American-cut suits are best for your shape (see page 109). A British-cut suit will also be fine as long as the fabric is soft (see page 107).

A loose-fitted jacket in a soft woven fabric is best.

Front-pleated trousers that sit as near to your waist as possible – braces (suspenders) will help. The best have a waistband with adjustments.

Your best fabrics

Flannel
Soft woven twill
Wool/Lycra mix
Wool and cashmere
Soft herringbone
Fabrics mixed with synthetics, such as Lycra

Your best patterns

Chalk stripes

Bird's eye

Pick and pick

Medium-weight tweed

Shirts

Fitted shirts will not work for you – a loose-fit shirt is your best option.

Your best fabrics

Cotton

Oxford cloth

Silk

Your best patterns

End to end

Herringbone

Ties

Choose patterns carefully and avoid horizontal stripes.

Your best fabrics

Plain or woven silk

Knitted

Your best patterns

Spots

Paisley

Floral

Soft geometric

Motifs

You should avoid

✗ Close-fitting jackets and shirts, trousers worn below the stomach, sharp tailoring and crisp fabrics.

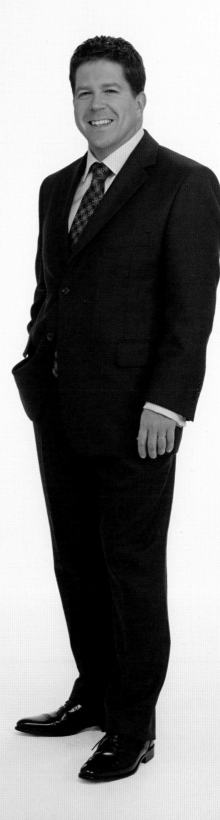

Rounded – casual wear

Comfort and correct fit are your priorities. Don't fall into the trap of allowing your casual trousers to slip further and further away from your natural waistline. This would give the illusion of shortening your legs and actually making your stomach look fuller. The target for you is not to add too much bulk in the way of clothes.

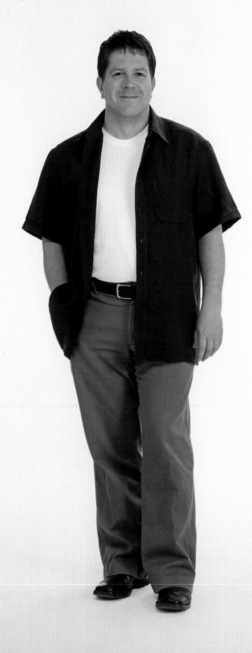

Your key rule

✓ Relaxed styling is the key to your casual look. A comfortable fit will ensure that your casual wardrobe remains flattering.

Jackets

Even if you prefer to wear it undone, make sure you can do up the jacket comfortably.

Your best styles
A deconstructed or dropped shoulder line jacket is a flattering style for your shape.

Substituting a shirt for a jacket is a great look for you.

Your best fabrics
Flannel
Wool and cashmere
Light- to medium-weight tweed
Linen
Suede
Fleece
Soft corduroy

Trousers

Make sure the pockets lie flat and the waistband sits straight and does not slip down.

Your best styles
Loose-fitting trousers with front pleats will be comfortable. Again, waist adjustments will add to the comfort.

Your best fabrics
Wool
Flannel
Cavalry twill
Soft denim
Chino
Parachute

Tops

If layering your clothes, choose lightweight fabrics to avoid bulk.

Your best styles
Make sure that loose-fitting tops don't swamp you.

Your best fabrics
Brushed cotton
Cotton
Knitted cotton
Medium-weight knits
Medium-weight jersey

Your best patterns

You can choose any subtle pattern within your colour palette.

You should avoid

✗ Clothing that is too loose or too tight; belted jackets and fitted tops, tight jeans and sharp geometric patterns.

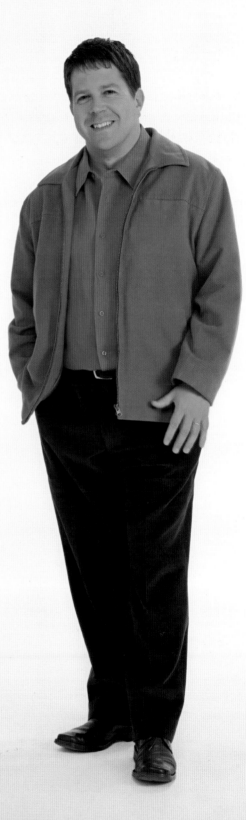

Your scale and height

Your scale is judged by the overall size of your skeleton and by features such as your nose, ears and mouth. Defined as fine, average or grand, your scale dictates the size of patterns, the weight of fabrics and the amount of texture that you can wear. Your scale will depend on various aspects of your build – see the boxes below to determine yours.

Understanding your scale

Your scale will be determined by your basic bone structure, this means the size of your wrists, hands and feet. Also, men with fine bone structures will normally have small facial features, so they will need to avoid heavyweight glasses and bulky knots in their ties. Conversely, a man with a large bone structure and a bigger facial figure will need to balance these with heavier weight frames, large knots in his tie and bulkier fabrics.

Note: There will be men who will be tall but fine in bone structure and others who will be short but have a heavier bone structure. Scale will dictate what you should wear.

Wearing colour for your height

Clever use of colour can make you appear taller or shorter; slimmer or fuller.

If you are short... If you are less than 1.68 m (5 ft 6 in) tall, you can make yourself appear taller by wearing the same colour trousers and top.

If you are of average height... If you measure between 1.68 and 1.83 m (5 ft 6 in–6 ft) tall any colour combination (see Chapter 2) will work well for you.

If you are tall... If you are more than 1.83 m (6 ft) tall, wearing different coloured tops and trousers will look more interesting on you. A darker top will make your torso look slimmer, while a lighter top will make your torso appear fuller.

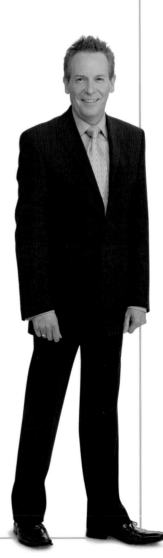

If you are fine scale...

You have
Small hands and feet
Small facial features
Small head

You should wear
Small patterns (for example, puppytooth as opposed to houndstooth)
Lightweight fabrics
Lightweight watches and belts

You should avoid
Bulky texture
Heavy, bulky shoes
Clothes that swamp you

Chest size
up to 97 cm (38 in)

Collar size
up to 37 cm (14½ in)

Your basic bone structure determines your scale — categorized as fine, average or grand — and this affects the size of patterns, the weight of fabrics and the amount of texture that you can wear.

If you are of average scale...

You have
A combination of sizes
Balanced facial features

You should wear
Medium-sized
patterns
Any weight of fabric
Appropriate
watches and belts

You should avoid
Tiny or overscale
patterns
Wearing bulky
layers

Chest size
97–112 cm (38–44 in)

Collar size
37–42 cm (14½–16½ in)

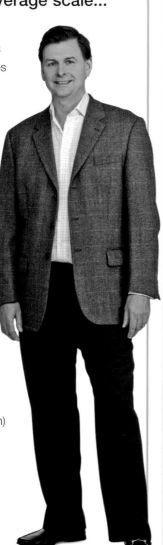

If you are grand scale...

You have
Large hands and feet
Large facial features
An impressive stature to your
appearance

You should wear
Larger patterns (for example,
houndstooth as opposed
to puppytooth)
Medium to heavy texture
Significant watches and
belts

You should avoid
Small patterns
Lightweight fabrics
Clothes that are too small

Chest size
over 112 cm (44 in)

Collar size
over 42 cm (16½ in)

Your proportions

One of the aspects of putting your clothes together is to understand your body's proportions – that is, the length of your body versus that of your legs. This will affect whether you tuck your casual shirts and other tops in, as well as the buttoning of your jacket in a formal suit.

Few men are completely in proportion. With off-the-peg suits, for example, if you buy a regular 107 cm (42 in) suit, the leg length is assumed to be 79 cm (31 in). However, most men do not fit neatly into these predetermined measurements. Some men's bodies are proportionally longer and hence their inside leg measurement shorter, and vice versa. This is why so many brands of suit trousers are available with unfinished hems or a choice of leg lengths. Similarly, you will find that jeans come in up to six different leg lengths for each waist measurement.

   To judge your proportions, stand in front of a mirror in your underwear and judge the position of your waist – it is roughly in line with your belly button. Then turn sideways and see whether your torso or your legs look longer (or whether they look balanced).

   Once you have discovered which category your body falls into, you will be able to follow a few simple guidelines to help you combine clothes and select colours and cuts that appear to adjust imbalances, resulting in a well-dressed style for all occasions.

Your natural waistline is roughly in line with your belly button.

Balanced...

Show-off your balanced proportions by:

✓ Wearing loose fitted tops tucked in to belted trousers

✓ Allowing fitted tops to hang loose

You should avoid:

✗ Wide trousers if you measure under 1.68 m (5 ft 6 in)

✗ Slim-fitting trousers if you measure over 1.83 m (6 ft)

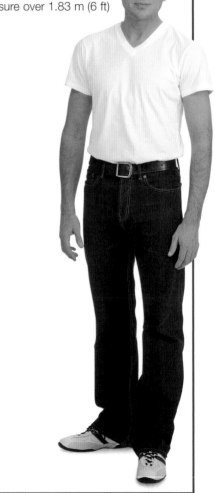

Short body and long legs...

Lower the appearance of your waistline by:

✓ Wearing your tops and shirts loose

✓ Opting for wider leg trousers

✓ Wearing trousers with turn-ups (cuffs)

✓ Choosing British-cut or Italian-style jackets (see pages 107–108)

✓ Wearing trousers with patterns and textures

You should avoid:

✗ Tucking in your casual shirts and tops

✗ High-buttoned/ short-collared jackets

✗ Tight-fitting slim-leg trousers

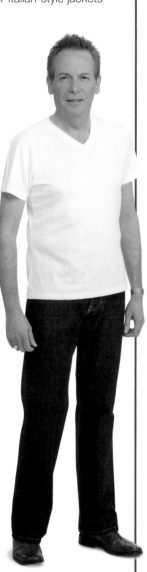

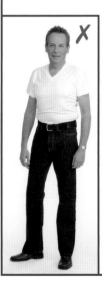

Long body and short legs...

Heighten the appearance of your waistline by:

✓ Wearing shorter length tops or tucking them in

✓ Opting for slim-line trousers

✓ Buttoning your jackets high

✓ Ensuring the colour of your top is lighter or brighter than that of your trousers

✓ Wearing suits, which creates a balanced look

You should avoid:

✗ Wide, baggy legged trousers

✗ Turn-ups (cuffs) on trousers if you are less than 1.83 m (6 ft)

✗ Long draping jackets

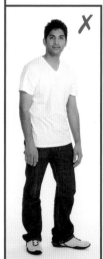

Balancing tricks

Not only can you enhance the appearance of your overall proportions (see pages 66–67) with clever clothing tricks, you can also alter the appearance of specific parts of your body to create the illusion of a near-perfect physique. Different colour combinations will make you look taller or shorter.

Your chest

Narrow chest

You are narrow chested if your chest is slightly hollowed. Your collar bones may be showing and your shoulders may be rounded. If this describes you, bear in mind the following:
Vertical stripes will give the illusion of width
Double-breasted jackets will look good on you
Layering will add bulk

Full chest

You may have a full or barrel chest if you have developed strong pectoral muscles through some form of weight training or regular exercise. Your chest will probably narrow down to your waist. You need to remember the following:
Horizontal stripes are slimming
Soft fabrics are better than crisp ones for you

Your arms

You will know whether your arms are longer or shorter than average if you have experienced problems with standard-fitting sleeves on clothes.

Long arms

If you have long arms wear:
Double (French) cuffs
Tops with a dropped shoulder line

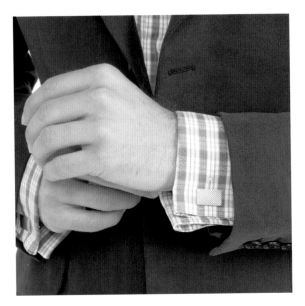

Short arms

If you have short arms you should:
Wear raglan sleeves
Adjust the sleeve length (see pages 116–119 on achieving a proper fit)
Ensure sleeves do not overhang your hands

Your shoulders

If you have sloping shoulders, avoid wearing raglan sleeves (sleeves without armhole seams, see page 141). If you have narrow shoulders, try wearing tops with a dropped shoulder line (where the shoulder seam is extended beyond the natural shoulder line and drops on to the upper arm).

Your neck

When you meet new people they invariably focus on your face first. Your face, your neck and what is worn around your neck are the overall focus of that first impression. You should therefore pay particular attention to the type of clothes that suit your neck.

Long neck

If you have a long neck you should wear:

Roll-necked sweaters

Nehru collars

Funnel necks

Crew-necks

Cut-away (spread) collars

Double Windsor tie knots

Bow ties

Short neck

If you have a short neck you should wear:

Open collared shirts

V-necks

Standard or long collar shirts

Half Windsor tie knots

Choosing a collar

When choosing a formal shirt, be aware that different collars have a different effect on your face and neckline. (See pages 146–147 to determine your face shape.)

Classic collar

Suits all face shapes and neck lengths.

Pointed collar

Best for rounded face shapes and wide necks.

Cutaway, or spread, collar

Good for narrow faces and long necks.

Button-down collar

For all face shapes. Can be worn with or without a tie.

Tab collar

Only for average to long necks.

Nehru collar

Best on a thin or long neck. If you have a short neck, wear it open.

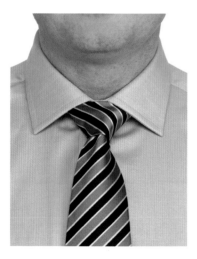

Standard collars suit all face shapes and necklines and will complement any tie knot.

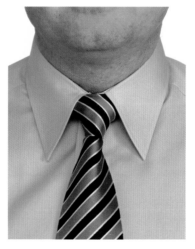

A pointed collar gives the illusion of narrowing and elongating the neck. Ensure that the knot balances with the collar.

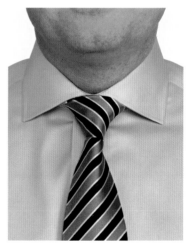

A widespread or cutaway collar has the effect of shortening and widening the neck.

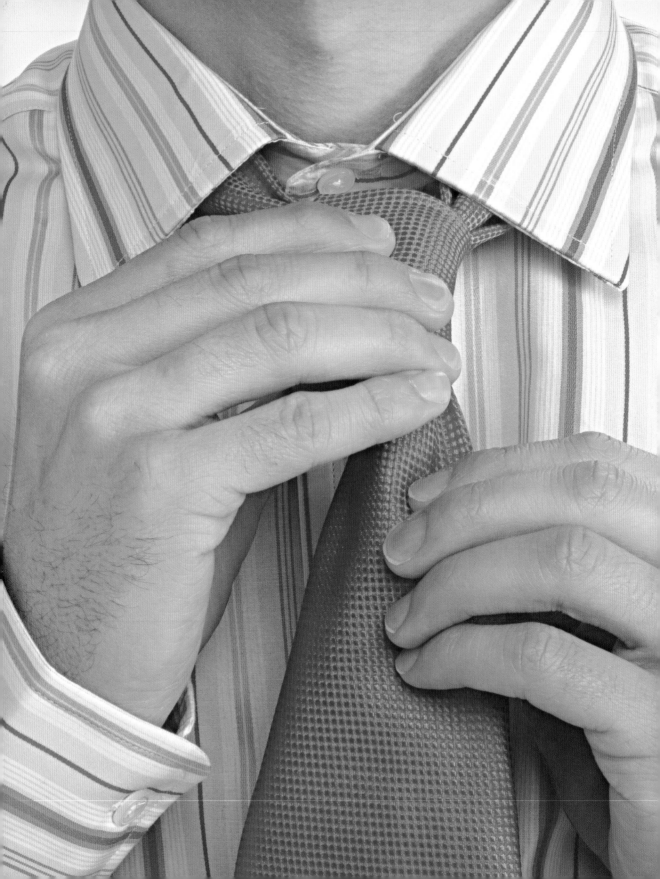

4

know yourself – know your style

Your 'signature'

You may think that now you know what colours to wear and what styles of clothes suit you, it's all over. However, whether you realize it or not, your personality and your attitude to your lifestyle, hobbies, cars and even the holidays you like to take, all have an impact on the clothes that you choose. This is your style personality, or 'signature'.

When taken out of our normal environment, with no dress code or uniform to adhere to, many of us feel lost. A sudden invitation to a weekend away, for example, may send you into a panic about what to wear. Understanding your signature will make you realize why you like to dress in a certain way. It will help you look at ease in whatever you choose to wear and also make putting your wardrobe together much easier and in a cohesive manner.

During your life there will be many influences – for example, age, lifestyle and budget – on your clothes, be they your school uniform or a dress code at work. Borrowing an idea from Shakespeare's well-known words on the seven ages of man makes it possible to demonstrate how the different stages of your life influence the way you dress.

The seven ages of man

1. Schoolboy
During this time of your life your upbringing has the major influence on your wardrobe. Your parents buy your clothes and you have little say in what you wear. You have no interest in how you look until your early teens when your individuality starts to show and you are subject to peer pressure.

2. College boy
Freedom at last! There is no one telling you to wash your hair, clean your shoes or even get out of bed. This is the time when you will probably be at your most creative in your style of dressing. Your wardrobe will be limited by your budget and you will probably be wearing what is clean at the time rather than what looks good on you.

'... one man in his time plays many parts, his acts being seven ages.' *As You Like It* William Shakespeare

3. Rake

Now you have started earning an income you have to make decisions on how to budget. For example, do you spend your money on what you wear to work, or do you spend it on what you wear at the weekends and out socializing? You may even start to look at men's magazines to consider the options and learn what is fashionable.

4. Lover

You now want to attract a partner and grooming will have become an important part of your daily routine. You are more likely to hang up your clothes at the end of the day, now that you have started to invest more in them. You might even consider that the colours you wear need to be less threatening and more approachable.

5. Parent

With the demands of parenthood, your income may once again be limited. In addition, your clothes may need to be more hardwearing and practical to withstand the traumas of messy babies and toddlers.

6. Businessman

With success now knocking at the door it is time for you to consider how others see you. Perhaps you'll want to think about spending a little more of your income on yourself and your wardrobe. Remember, your body may not be in the same shape as it once was.

7. Retirement age

Retirement brings the opportunity to be the real you without the constraints of considering what to wear to work. For many men, this can be a formidable challenge. By understanding your personal look, you will have defined guidelines to help you.

All your life experiences will have influenced your style and you need to ensure that this look is now completed rather than being a mishmash of many different stages in your life.

Identify your style

By completing the style personality questionnaire overleaf you will be able to identify a trend in your personal preferences – from Creative to International. You can then develop this trend into your personal look. This information will provide you – and those who shop for you – with a theme and a focus that you can carry throughout your wardrobe for all occasions.

Style personality questionnaire

A good image means expressing your personality and being comfortable with how you dress whether you are at work, at home or socializing. Answer the following questions as honestly as you can, by selecting as many choices as you feel appropriate. Your style personality will be the catalyst in bringing your whole wardrobe together.

How would you describe your overall look?

- [ ] **A** Eclectic and sometimes crazy
- [ ] **B** Different – I like to make an entrance
- [ ] **C** Thought through and coordinated
- [ ] **D** Traditional
- [ ] **E** Relaxed
- [ ] **F** Understated but well groomed

What do you wear for work?

- [ ] **A** Something different every day
- [ ] **B** Clothes that make a statement
- [ ] **C** Clothes that are elegant
- [ ] **D** Conservative, never overstated, clothes
- [ ] **E** Comfortable clothes
- [ ] **F** Current, but not high-fashion, clothes

What do you wear at the weekend?

- [ ] **A** I like to put things together in an unusual way
- [ ] **B** My latest buys
- [ ] **C** I like texture and interesting fabrics
- [ ] **D** Smart casual
- [ ] **E** Combats and a t-shirt
- [ ] **F** Smart jeans and a polo shirt

What is your favourite jacket?

- [ ] **A** One I found abroad or at a market
- [ ] **B** A designer one
- [ ] **C** A velvet one
- [ ] **D** A navy blazer
- [ ] **E** A fleece
- [ ] **F** A fitted sports jacket

What are your favourite shoes?

- [ ] **A** Boots
- [ ] **B** My newest shoes
- [ ] **C** Ones with tassels
- [ ] **D** Brogues
- [ ] **E** Trainers
- [ ] **F** Slip-on loafers

How would you describe your tie collection?

- [ ] **A** Lots of different designs, including bow ties
- [ ] **B** Striking and bold colour combinations
- [ ] **C** My ties tell a story
- [ ] **D** Good quality and matching my shirts
- [ ] **E** I don't have a collection, just a couple of ties for special occasions
- [ ] **F** I update it regularly

A good image means expressing your personality and being comfortable with how you dress whether you are at work, relaxing at the weekend or out socializing.

What do you wear for a night out on the town?

- ☐ **A** Whatever catches my eye
- ☐ **B** Something unique-looking
- ☐ **C** A silk shirt and smart trousers
- ☐ **D** A blazer and flannel trousers
- ☐ **E** A sweater and jeans
- ☐ **F** A linen suit

What would your favourite holiday be?

- ☐ **A** Somewhere I have never been before
- ☐ **B** Action-packed
- ☐ **C** A long weekend in Venice
- ☐ **D** I like to return to places I know
- ☐ **E** Walking and hiking
- ☐ **F** A place with some culture

What are your thoughts on grooming products?

- ☐ **A** I use natural products when I think about it
- ☐ **B** I use products on my hair
- ☐ **C** I like to test new products
- ☐ **D** I use them when I need to
- ☐ **E** They are not a priority
- ☐ **F** I have a good skincare routine

What is your dream car?

- ☐ **A** Original Beetle/2 CV
- ☐ **B** Lexus sport/Ferrari
- ☐ **C** Classic or vintage
- ☐ **D** Mercedes/Jaguar
- ☐ **E** Estate car
- ☐ **F** Mini Cooper S/Audi TT

Once you have completed the questionnaire, count how many times you have answered A, B, C, etc. You can then determine your predominant style below and refer to the appropriate pages to read more about your personal look.

Mainly A	Creative	*see pages 76–77*
Mainly B	Dramatic	*see pages 78–79*
Mainly C	Romantic	*see pages 80–81*
Mainly D	Classic	*see pages 82–83*
Mainly E	Natural	*see pages 84–85*
Mainly F	International	*see pages 86–87*

Creative

You have an individual look, which varies from day to day. You do not enjoy shopping in a shopping mall – you prefer to visit one-off boutiques, market stalls or even second-hand stores. You may feel challenged in a formal business environment but as long as your look is appropriate you need not lose your creative input into your wardrobe.

Famous Creatives

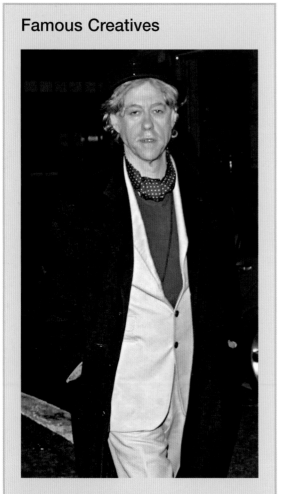

Sir Bob Geldof (pictured)
David Bowie
Sir Elton John
John Galliano

Lifestyle

✓ You tend to like creative hobbies like painting, music and writing.

✓ You are a collector.

✓ You prefer public transport to any other methods of getting you from A to B.

Style characteristics

✓ Your wardrobe consists of one-off pieces.

✓ You like to stroll around markets and buy whatever catches your eye.

✓ You can still be creative in a formal environment through your choice of ties, cufflinks and colour combinations.

✓ You may colour your hair for effect and to be different, and wear it in a textured, loose style.

Make the most of your style...

✓ Try mixing and matching your fabrics, for example, stripes and checks.

✓ Mix formal and casual wear together.

✓ Add interesting accessories.

✓ Combine vintage or retro-style clothes with new ones.

Make the most of your colours...

	Formal		Casual	
	Suit	Shirt	Trousers	Shirt
Light	pewter	sage	light teal	blush pink
Deep	chocolate	taupe	royal purple	scarlet
Warm	bronze	primrose	stone	turquoise
Cool	pine	icy green	dark denim	purple
Clear	black brown	light peach	light grey	Chinese blue
Muted	grey green	sage	soft violet	claret

Accessories

✓ A fob watch would be your first choice.

✓ Seek out interesting buckles for your belts from markets or boutiques.

✓ A Gladstone bag is perfect for you.

✓ For shoes, try interesting colours and materials. Try teaming fashion trainers with suits.

Grooming

✓ Because your look is unusual take care not to give the impression that you are not well groomed (see Chapter 7).

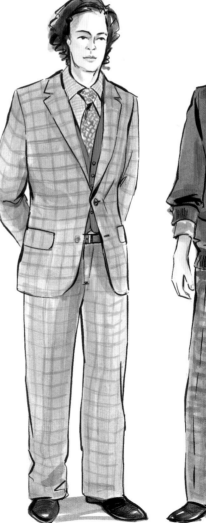
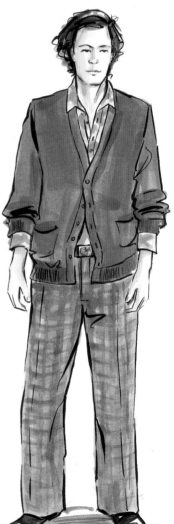

Dramatic

You love to shop and buy the latest fashions and gadgets. Regardless of your colouring you like bold and strong colour statements. You probably change your hairstyle often, making use of all the latest grooming products available. In very formal environments you may have to tone down your exuberance and your desire to be flamboyant.

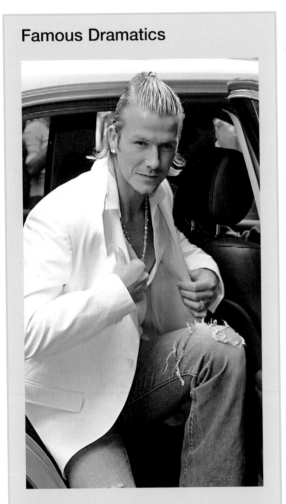

Famous Dramatics

David Beckham (pictured)
Robbie Williams
P. Diddy
George Michael

Lifestyle

✓ You like to drive fast cars and perhaps take the odd risk or two.

✓ You like sports that call for specialized equipment.

✓ Your home is full of the latest hi-tech gadgets.

Style characteristics

✓ Your wardrobe is brimming with wonderful statement pieces.

✓ You research the internet and magazines for shopping ideas.

✓ You can outshine your partner when the pair of you are dressed for socializing.

✓ Practicality doesn't enter your mind when you are out shopping.

Make the most of your style...

✓ Don't get carried away and buy a one-off garment that won't go with anything else in your wardrobe.

✓ Wear colour for effect.

✓ Ensure you change the style of your jackets and suits periodically.

✓ Have shoes or boots to go with all your looks.

Make the most of your colours...

	Formal		Casual	
	Suit	**Shirt**	**Trousers**	**Shirt**
Light	medium charcoal	violet	cream	geranium
Deep	black	icy violet	navy	lime
Warm	chocolate	oatmeal	terracotta	medium denim
Cool	dark navy	rose pink	sapphire	duck egg
Clear	light grey	medium grey	chocolate	apple green
Muted	charcoal	claret	medium denim	light periwinkle

Accessories

✓ Wear a chronometer rather than a watch.

✓ Make sure the statement buckle on your belt doesn't overpower your look.

✓ You should have nothing less than a designer-label bag.

✓ Wear shoes with a difference.

Grooming

✓ Make sure you use all the grooming products you bought just to get the designer-label bag.

✓ If you have tattoos it might be appropriate to conceal them in a formal environment.

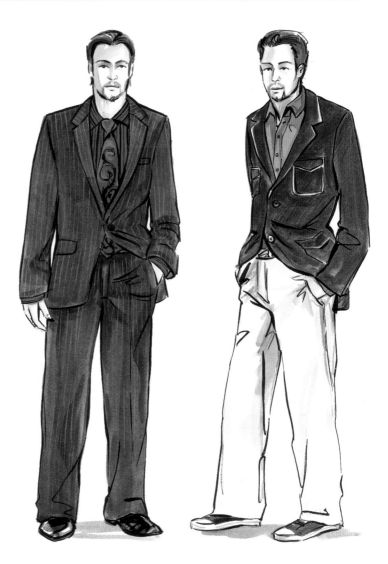

Romantic

You have a sense of security in your look and are not afraid to make others aware of your interest in looking after yourself. You enjoy shopping but think a purchase through before buying it. You care about your grooming and invest time and money in it. You like interesting fabrics that are often luxurious.

Famous Romantics

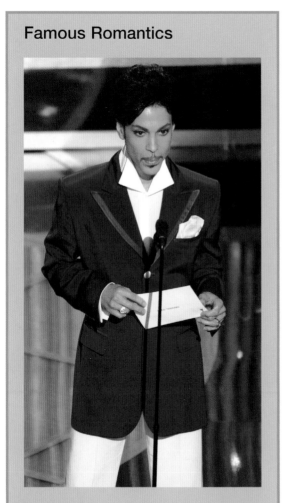

Prince (pictured)
Donald Trump
Bryan Ferry
Sting

Lifestyle

✓ You have a regular exercise regime to keep yourself fit and healthy.

✓ You like luxurious and comfortable modes of travel.

✓ You care about your environment whether at home or at work.

Style characteristics

✓ Your clothes are well maintained, and are pressed and hung up at the end of the day.

✓ You like to shop where you know you will get good service and advice.

✓ You are always appropriately dressed for every occasion – formal or informal.

✓ For you, in order to get it right, it's all in the detail.

Make the most of your style...

✓ Think luxury fabrics and texture, like cashmere, tweed and washable silk.

✓ Choose your suits carefully to fit your body shape (see Chapter 3).

✓ Consider wearing double (French) cuffs with silk knots for your casual wear.

✓ Treat yourself to either a velvet or a suede jacket.

Make the most of your colours...

	Formal		Casual	
	Suit	**Shirt**	**Trousers**	**Shirt**
Light	taupe	cream	peacock	light teal
Deep	charcoal	icy violet	dark denim	true blue
Warm	olive	grey green	terracotta	tangerine
Cool	spruce	icy green	charcoal	light grey
Clear	dark navy	sky blue	cornflower	Chinese blue
Muted	pewter	shell	sage	verbena

Accessories

✓ You have a collection of watches to wear for different occasions.

✓ You have belts in different colours and weights of leather.

✓ You carry your papers around in a thin portfolio case.

✓ You never fail to wear the right shoes for your look, whatever the occasion.

Grooming

✓ Be willing to wear your hair shorter once it starts thinning.

✓ Make sure your aftershave stays with you, and doesn't remain behind after you have left the room.

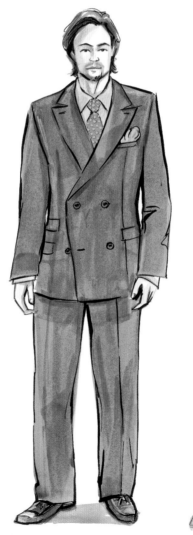
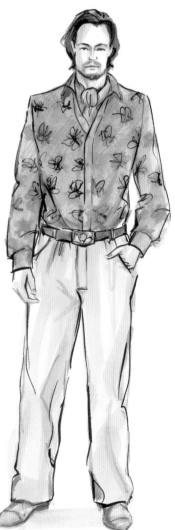

Classic

You are a man of tradition, you are comfortable with your look and see no reason to change it. You don't like taking risks, particularly with your clothes. You are well coordinated and rarely experiment with different colour combinations. When presented with something new, however, you can be open minded.

Famous Classics

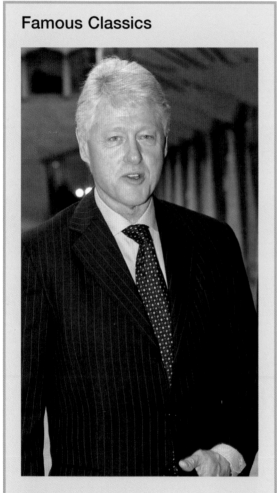

Bill Clinton (pictured)
Prince Charles
Colin Powell
King Juan Carlos

Lifestyle

✓ You like your hobbies and sports to be structured and timed, for example, golf and tennis.

✓ Once you find your favourite car, you tend to stick to the same model.

✓ Whether it's a desk or garden shed, you keep your work area organized.

Style characteristics

✓ Your wardrobe is neat and tidy.

✓ You shop only when necessary and in stores that you know.

✓ Even in your casual clothes, you have an air of tradition and formality.

✓ You rarely change your hairstyle.

Make the most of your style...

✓ Don't be afraid to experiment with colour or shape of clothes.

✓ Be aware that fashion changes for men about once a decade (for example the width of ties and jacket lapels) and you need to update your wardrobe.

✓ Experiment with your casual look – try jeans and a sweater for a change.

Make the most of your colours...

	Formal			Casual	
	Suit	**Shirt**		**Trousers**	**Shirt**
Light	light navy	ivory		taupe	sky blue
Deep	dark navy	soft white		charcoal	burgundy
Warm	charcoal	cream		grey green	teal
Cool	medium grey	sky blue		dark denim	bluebell
Clear	dark navy	light peach		black	true blue
Muted	charcoal blue	sky blue		rose brown	verbena

Accessories

✓ You wear the watch you were given for a special occasion.

✓ You may need to consider a casual belt for your casual trousers.

✓ You carry a briefcase whatever you put in it.

✓ You look after your shoes so that they last well.

Grooming

✓ Update your hairstyle once in a while and try a different stylist.

✓ Don't be afraid to use appropriate hair and skincare products (see pages 149–153) – they will make a difference.

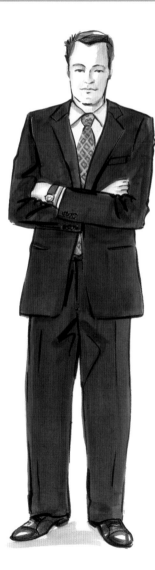
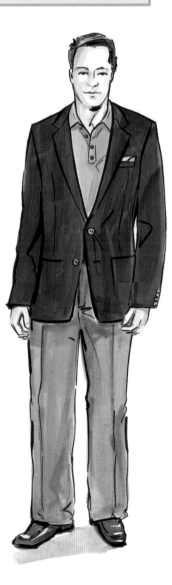

Natural

You have a very relaxed attitude to virtually everything; you are the typical laid-back man. You like your clothes to be comfortable and easy to look after. If you are ever forced to wear a jacket and tie, the jacket spends most of its time on a hook, with the tie loose around your neck. You are the one who struggles the most with formal business wear.

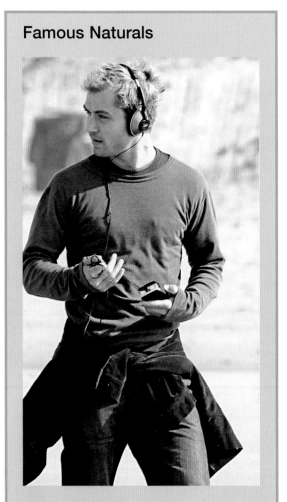

Famous Naturals

Jude Law (pictured)
Bill Gates
Jamie Oliver
Richard Branson

Lifestyle

✓ You are into sports of all kinds, whether you participate in them or just watch.

✓ Your chosen mode of transport is functional rather than stylish.

✓ You have a relaxed attitude to the décor of your home environment.

Style characteristics

✓ Your wardrobe consists of comfortable clothes that don't coordinate.

✓ You simply don't like shopping.

✓ You find grooming a chore.

✓ Your hair tends to be longer than most and you may sport designer stubble.

Make the most of your style...

✓ Clothes maintenance needs to become part of your routine.

✓ Deconstructed and loose-fitting clothes give you a relaxed look.

✓ A jacket and trousers combination is always your preferred business look but, for a formal work environment, consider the amazing washable business suit that is now widely available.

Make the most of your colours...

	Formal		Casual	
	Suit	**Shirt**	**Trousers**	**Shirt**
Light	medium charcoal	soft white	light denim	light teal
Deep	dark navy	mint	dark denim	burgundy
Warm	charcoal	cream	medium denim	terracotta
Cool	dark navy	icy blue	dark denim	sapphire
Clear	black	ivory	dark denim	evergreen
Muted	light navy	sky blue	medium denim	jade

Accessories

✓ You will want a multi-functional watch – make sure it doesn't overpower your scale (see pages 64–65).

✓ If your trousers have belt loops you need to wear a belt to complete the look.

✓ Depending on your job, a rucksack type of bag may be your preference.

✓ Your shoes need to be comfortable but ensure that they are appropriate for the rest of your look (see pages 124–125).

Grooming

✓ Try to make having a haircut a regular part of your life. Every five or six weeks is the rule, and don't forget to make your next appointment before you leave.

✓ For an easy life, choose clothes that are low maintenance (for example easy-iron shirts and stretch jeans) and fabrics containing Lycra, which return to their original shape. Try to remember to hang up your clothes at the end of the day.

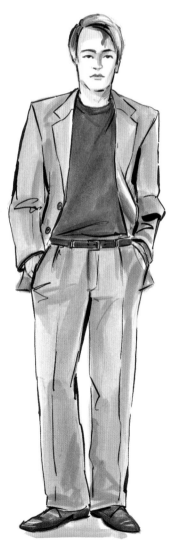
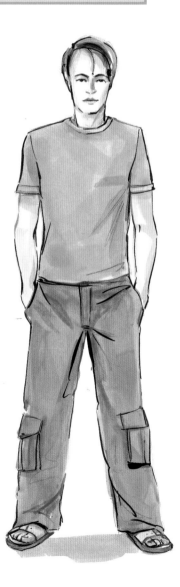

International

You may feel that you are a little bit of all the other looks. This is the true International look – adapting your style to suit your location and the occasion. You are adept at changing a shirt or a tie to completely alter your look. Even though your budget may be limited, you buy wisely to ensure that you have a coordinated wardrobe.

Famous Internationals

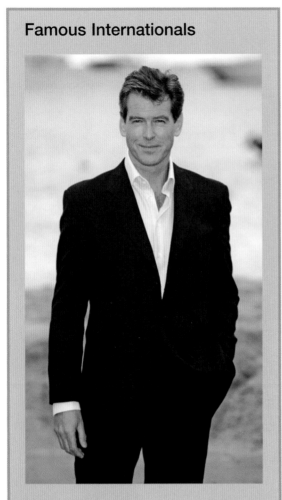

Pierce Brosnan (pictured)
George Clooney
Kofi A. Annan
Johnny Depp

Lifestyle

✓ You choose a sport that can be pursued anywhere in the world, be it tennis or swimming.

✓ Your car of choice would be trendy but not ostentatious.

✓ You are a minimalist in both your home and your work environment.

Style characteristics

✓ You add shirts and other tops to update your core wardrobe.

✓ You know what you want when you go shopping and are prepared to look for it.

✓ You care about your grooming but you are not a fanatic. You prefer to spend your money on dental care rather than on a fast car.

✓ You are confident about letting your hair go naturally grey and thin.

Make the most of your style...

✓ Don't wear extreme colour combinations, you will feel more comfortable in neutral colours.

✓ Update your formal look with new ties.

✓ Learn about the latest trends by consulting newspapers and magazines.

Make the most of your colours...

	Formal		Casual	
	Suit	**Shirt**	**Trousers**	**Shirt**
Light	taupe	mint	light denim	light periwinkle
Deep	dark navy	icy violet	aubergine	royal purple
Warm	chocolate	buttermilk	sage	grey green
Cool	medium grey	icy grey	dark denim	light teal
Clear	charcoal	sky blue	stone	emerald turquoise
Muted	pewter	ivory	natural beige	sage

Accessories

✓ Have three watches: one for daytime, evening and sports.

✓ Coordinate the colour of your belts with those of your shoes.

✓ Invest in good-quality shoes.

Grooming

✓ Change your hairdresser/barber so that your hairstyle gets updated.

✓ Experiment with aftershaves to find one you like.

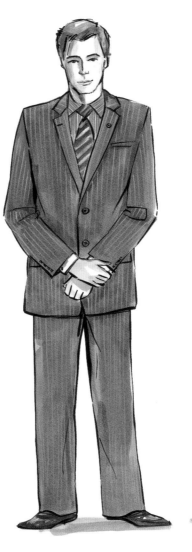
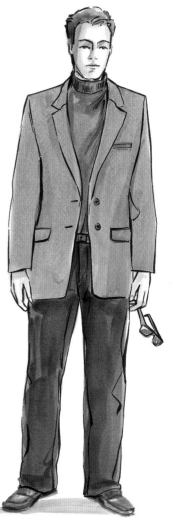

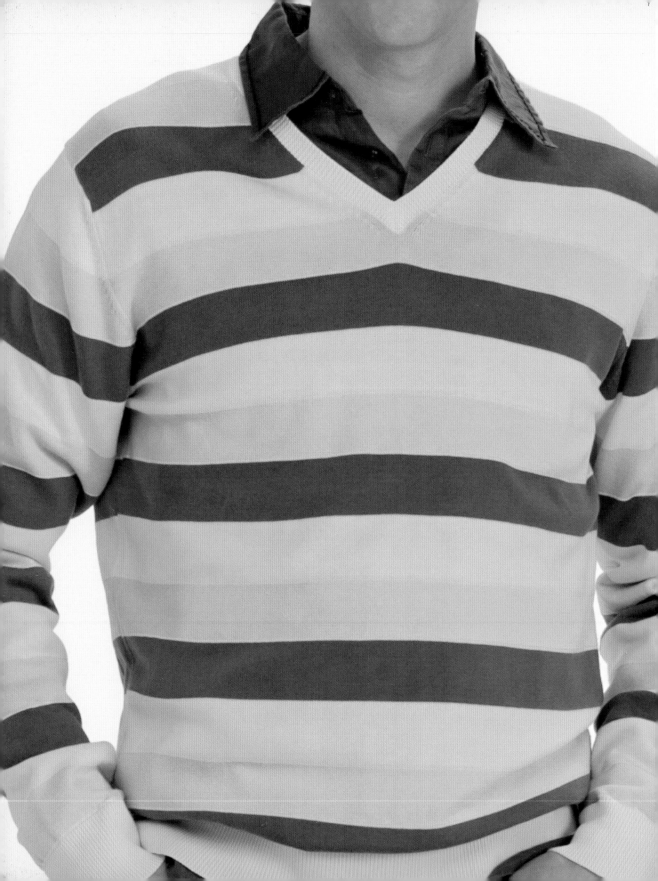

5

looking the part

Conveying your message

Having discovered your best colours, found out about your build and your personal look, you now need to ensure that your look is appropriate for wherever you are going. One of the elements of being well dressed is being appropriately dressed for every occasion, circumstance, locality and age group. There are also cultural differences which you need to consider. Sometimes you may think that as long as your clothes are clean, 'it'll do'. But the way you put your look together will send different messages to those around you.

There are occasions when a suit and tie are the only appropriate attire. Conversely, you might be regarded as overdressed in that same suit and tie when the rest of the group is casually dressed. With the trend for more casual work environments, don't be afraid to ask about the dress code before starting a new job.

This chapter provides you with general guidelines for appropriate dressing for different scenarios. Don't assume, nowadays, that you have to wear a suit to attend a wedding; likewise don't take it for granted that you can go to a party in jeans.

Product 'you'

When meeting new people for the first time, you need to think about what first impression your look will convey. When launching any new product, the manufacturers think about its placement in the market and how it will be displayed.

Think of yourself as a product and consider what messages your image is conveying about you.

Your image

If you want be seen as...	Think about...
friendly and approachable	colour
relaxed	comfort
creative	looking different
innovative	being current
knowledgeable	maturity
efficient	grooming
professional	business dress
international	the style of your clothes
a leader	looking inspiring

For example, the styling of the VW Beetle has been updated to keep up with current technologies, but the classic lines are still there, while Renault is innovative in its design lines and constantly changing the basic shape of its mainstream models. In the same way, think of yourself as a product and choose your clothes according to where you are going that day and who you are going to meet, and decide what non-verbal messages you want your appearance to convey about yourself (see box, opposite).

Appropriate dress

Nothing can be more embarrassing than arriving at a job interview or social gathering and being inappropriately dressed. You may be somebody who has a Natural style personality and find it challenging to dress formally if an occasion calls for it; you might also offend your hosts and feel totally out of place. Conversely, as a Classic invited to a barbecue, a navy blazer, cravat and calvary twill trousers will be totally over the top.

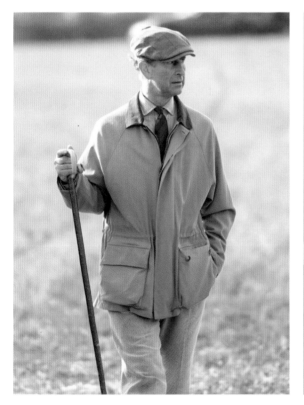

Prince Charles has a vast wardrobe to suit every occasion and always appears appropriately dressed.

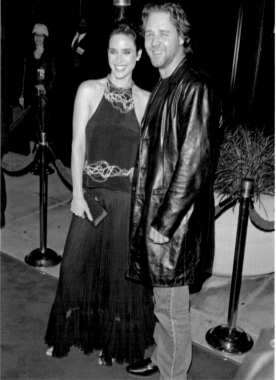

Russell Crowe let his partner down badly by wearing jeans and a leather jacket to this premiere.

Interview success

If you are going for a job interview where you and the other candidates are equally well qualified, you want to ensure that your image helps you win that interview rather than damage your chances. First of all, consider the industry you want to work in. Is there a strict dress code? Research the company and find out what their branding values are. Next, you need to decide what to wear – dress for the interview as if you are already a member of the team.

What to wear

Your clothes need to be unmemorable and understated so, whether formal or casual, neutral colours are safest. If a tie is called for, this is where you can add some colour, but it must coordinate with your shirt and jacket.

Grooming

✓ Make sure your hair is trimmed and clean but don't look as though you have just come from the hairdresser/barber.

✓ Long hair needs to be tied back.

✓ If you wear a beard or moustache make sure it is trimmed.

✓ Unruly eyebrows, nose and ear hair need to be plucked and tamed.

✓ Fingernails must be clean – if you are a nail biter, have a manicure beforehand.

✓ Use a mouth freshener before going into the interview room.

✓ If your interview is at the end of the day, you will need a clean shirt and socks to ensure you are fresh looking.

✓ Avoid the '5 o'clock shadow' look.

Accessories

✓ Wear understated accessories – no chronometers or Mickey Mouse watches.

✓ Your shoes need to be appropriate for your clothes, and must be clean. Check for worn-out heels and driver's scuff marks.

✓ Your socks should be free of logos and tone with your trousers and shoes.

✓ If there are loops on your trouser waistband, you need to wear a belt – make sure it is an appropriate colour and style for your trousers.

✓ Papers need to be kept in a folder – leave rucksacks and big bags at reception. If taking notes, make sure you have a decent pen.

Body language

Keep your body language open and relaxed. Closed hand movements and crossed arms give the impression of being defensive. By sitting comfortably with your back against the chair you will look confident. Keep your body facing the interviewer and if angling your position make it towards the interviewer. As a primate we have the unconscious ability to analyse body language. Taking a little time to be aware of others and your own body language will give you that extra edge.

Eye contact

Good eye contact is essential during an interview, although staring at somebody intensely over a long time can be very off-putting. If you find eye contact difficult, try talking to the interviewer's left or right ear. Dark tinted glasses should not be worn.

How you sound

Although you may be nervous, try and speak slowly. If you find that difficult, use pauses to help you pace what you are saying. Deep breathing while waiting will also help you relax.

Handshake

Get a friend to check your handshake to ensure that it is neither the wet fish nor the knuckle crusher. A good handshake should be vertically palm to palm, with a firm grip, while maintaining eye contact.

Things to avoid...

✗ Don't wear bright and garish clothes and colours, even in a creative environment.

✗ Avoid using too much aftershave – you don't want to be the candidate remembered for the lingering smell.

✗ Be sure not to consume curries, alcohol, coffee and tobacco before an interview, as they can all taint your breath and stain your teeth.

Formal business meeting

Whether you are attending an internal or external formal meeting, take steps with your appearance to maximize your effectiveness. Both the climate and the industry you work in will obviously dictate the correct mode of dress, the former influencing the weight and the colour of the fabrics for your business suit. If working in the tropics, for example, you will want lighter-weight fabrics in the lighter shades of the neutrals in your colour palette.

Using colours

Appropriate colour combinations can alter people's perception of you. Depending on your role in the meeting – as leader or participant – follow these colour guidelines to look the part.

If you are heading the meeting – the leader – use colour combinations that give you control and authority: a dark suit, light shirt and contrasting tie.

If you are involved as a participant in the discussion or brain-storming, you need less authoritative colours. The colours need to convey openness instead.

Jacket on or off?

When attending a meeting take the lead from the chairperson as to whether you can take off your jacket and loosen your tie. If you do, note the following:

✓ Your shirt must be tucked in properly.

✓ There can be no sweat marks on your shirt.

Leader

Light
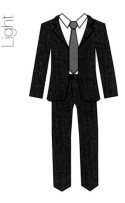
suit: light navy
shirt: ivory
tie: geranium

Deep
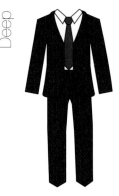
suit: dark navy
shirt: soft white
tie: burgundy

Warm
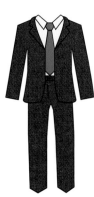
suit: charcoal
shirt: cream
tie: bittersweet

Cool
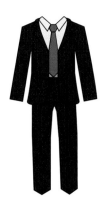
suit: dark navy
shirt: icy blue
tie: blue-red

Clear
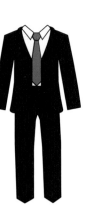
suit: dark navy
shirt: soft white
tie: scarlet

Muted
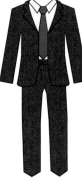
suit: charcoal
shirt: ivory
tie: claret

✓ Don't wear a lightweight shirt if you have a hairy chest – it will show through the fine fabric – and try to avoid loosening your top button, too.

✓ Never wear short sleeves under a suit. If it is warm you can roll up your shirt sleeves.

The climate and industry in which you work will, to some extent, dictate your mode of dress.

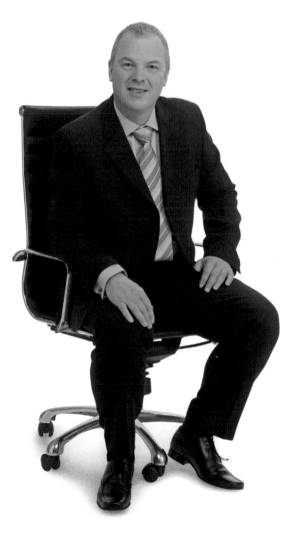

Participant

Light

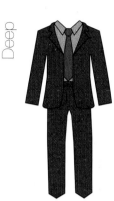

suit: pewter
shirt: cream
tie: sage

Deep

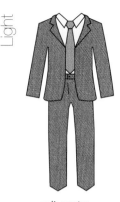

suit: chocolate
shirt: taupe
tie: forest

Warm

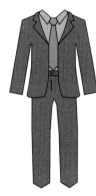

suit: bronze
shirt: stone
tie: terracotta

Cool

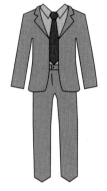

suit: medium grey
shirt: light grey
tie: charcoal

Clear

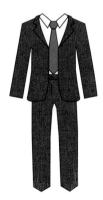

suit: charcoal
shirt: ivory
tie: cornflower

Muted

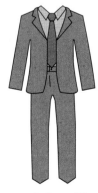

suit: charcoal blue
shirt: sky blue
tie: light navy

Business casual dress code

In many industries and professions, business casual is now the norm. It is a relaxed style of dressing that is still professional, but comfortable, mixing casual elements with smarter basics.

There are many options for adopting the business casual style. You can relax a formal suit by wearing it with a soft collared shirt and no tie; a polo shirt or a polo-necked sweater might also be a good alternative. Consider a sports jacket or simply wear a smart shirt with casual trousers and a more adventurous tie. Swap your formal brogues for easy slip-on loafers.

Fine-tuning your look

Creative Combine a windowpane tweed jacket and checked shirt with corduroy trousers.

Dramatic A black linen suit with a grey twill shirt.

Romantic A corduroy jacket, chambray shirt and lightweight wool trousers.

Classic Try a blazer, a button-down collar shirt and cavalry twill trousers.

Natural Opt for an unlined jacket, soft-collared shirt and chinos for a relaxed look.

International Looks good in a houndstooth jacket and silk-and-linen-mix trousers and Oxford cloth shirt.

Remember...

✓ Your grooming is important.

✓ Avoid the following casual styles: trainers or flip-flops (thongs); t-shirts; combats; jeans; Lycra.

Inverted triangle

Jackets
Blazer (double-breasted)
Sports jacket in fine tweed of houndstooth/puppytooth
Suit

Shirts
Button-down collar
Twill
Soft collar
Formal worn without jacket

Tops
Polo shirt
Roll-neck sweater in fine wool

Trousers
Flat-fronted tailored chinos

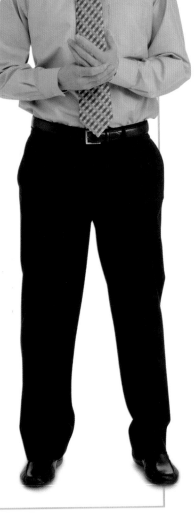

The Rectangle

Jackets
Blazer (single-breasted)
Fitted sports jacket in
tweed or houndstooth
Linen suit

Shirts
Button-down collar
Soft collar
Short-sleeved
Formal worn
without jacket

Tops
Polo shirt
Roundneck
sweater in
wool

Trousers
Flat-fronted
tailored
chinos

The Rounded

Jackets
Linen suit
Soft wool sports (single- or double-breasted)

Shirts
Button-down collar
Soft collar

Tops
Polo shirt
V-neck sweater in
fine wool

Trousers
Pleated-front
tailored
moleskin

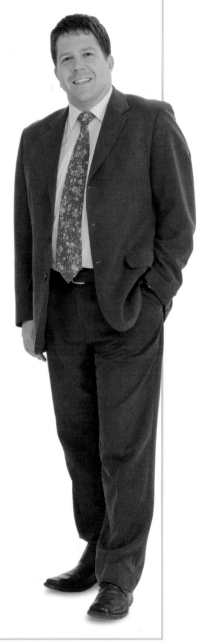

Smart casual dress code

Smart casual is a relaxed way of dressing for an occasion in which you can feel comfortable and yet still be appropriately dressed. With so many calls for a 'smart casual' dress code – an away day from the office, a family reunion or an evening out – the boundaries are flexible.

A smart casual wardrobe does not only consist of a pair of jeans and a couple of t-shirts – you should also include some of the following: a casual jacket, button-down collar or soft-collar shirts, cords or smart jeans, v-neck sweaters or polo shirts. Consider the occasion carefully – your choice of clothes for an outdoor event will differ from those for a formal family lunch.

Fine-tuning your look

Creative Try a vintage jacket with a waistcoat (vest) and silk shirt.
Dramatic Combine a black leather jacket with a black shirt and designer-label jeans.
Romantic A velvet jacket, pink shirt and wool trousers would work well for you.
Classic Opt for a blazer, twill shirt and flannel trousers.
Natural Try a tweed jacket, polo shirt and chinos.
International Combining a sports jacket, roll-neck sweater and twill trousers creates a timeless look.

Remember...

✓ Your accessories should be complementary.

✓ Wear the right footwear (see pages 124–125).

Inverted triangle

Jackets
Shaped sports jacket in crisp fabric or leather
Linen and silk
Lightweight tweed

Shirts
Short-sleeved
Nehru
Collarless
Denim

Tops
Rugby shirt
Fitted t-shirt
Crew neck
Raglan v-neck

Trousers
Flat-fronted
Smart jeans
Chinos
Cords

The Rectangle

Jackets
Casual coat
Cotton
Corduroy

Shirts
Button-down collar
Soft collar with
breast pocket
Short-sleeved
Cheesecloth
(muslin)

Tops
Rugby shirt
Polo shirt
Standard t-shirt
V-neck sweater

Trousers
Flat-fronted
Smart jeans
Chinos

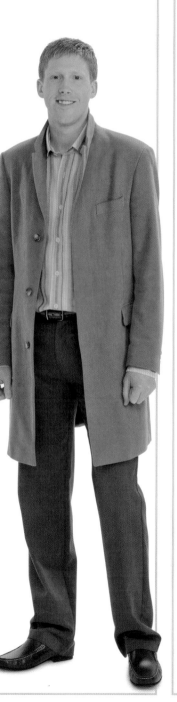

The Rounded

Jackets
Blouson
Flannel blazer (double-breasted)
Soft wool sports

Shirts
Button-down collar
Soft collar with breast pocket
Short-sleeved

Tops
Plain rugby shirt
Polo shirt
Loose t-shirt
V-neck sweater

Trousers
Pleated-fronted
Soft-styled jeans
Chinos
Cords

Dress right for the night

There will be occasions when you are called to wear 'black tie'. This is a classic look which has to be followed to the letter if the occasion is very formal. If the event is lower key, however, some personalization is acceptable. If you don't own a dress suit, you could hire one or wear the darkest suit that you own, with a white shirt and a dark tie.

The jacket

Black tuxedo The standard black tuxedo jacket is unvented (see 'Vents', page 106).
White tuxedo This is traditionally worn at open-air evening events or on board cruise ships.

Your body shape (see pages 50–51) will dictate the best style of jacket for you:
Inverted triangle Peaked lapel (either single- or double-breasted)
Rectangle Notched lapel (single-breasted)
Rounded Shawl collar (single-breasted)

The waistcoat (vest) and cummerbund

You have the option of wearing a waistcoat (vest) (although not with a double-breasted jacket) or cummerbund.

Inverted triangle Waistcoat (vest) or cummerbund.
Rectangle Waistcoat (vest) or cummerbund.
Rounded Waistcoat (vest) only.

The dress shirt

Collar A regular collar works for everyone. A wing collar is best on men with long necks and with single-breasted jackets with peaked lapels. The bow tie should be worn in front of the wing-collar tabs, not tucked behind them.
Shirt front The shirt will either be fly-fronted or allow for two or three studs (the number traditionally depends upon the wearer's height). The front of a dress shirt is reinforced so as to allow the wearer to sit down without the shirt bulging up. The trimming, usually pleats or pique (or reinforced cotton) does not go as low as the waistband.
Cuffs The traditional dress shirt always has double (French) cuffs.

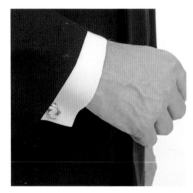
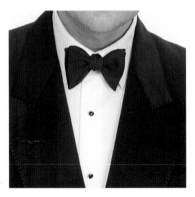
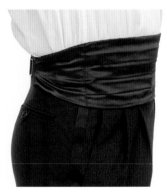

The tie

If the dress code is 'black tie', you should wear a black bow tie that you tie yourself (see page 123). If the event is less formal, you can have fun by wearing a coloured silk evening bow tie.

The trousers

The outside seam of dress trousers are embellished with a silk stripe. They have no turn-ups (cuffs) and are worn with braces (suspenders) or have self-adjustments – never wear a belt with them.

The shoes

Ideally, you will have some black patent leather evening shoes, although the majority of men opt for a highly polished pair of Oxfords (see pages 124–125).

Velvet jacket

The velvet jacket evolved from the smoking jacket and it is now acceptable on less formal occasions to wear a dark velvet jacket. This could be worn with one of the following combinations:

✓ A dress shirt with an untied bow tie or with no bow tie at all

✓ A silk shirt, with or without an evening tie

✓ A Nehru shirt

Remember…

✓ Always be freshly shaved for the occasion

✓ Take a clean handkerchief (to dab away the perspiration if dancing!)

✓ Wear only black socks

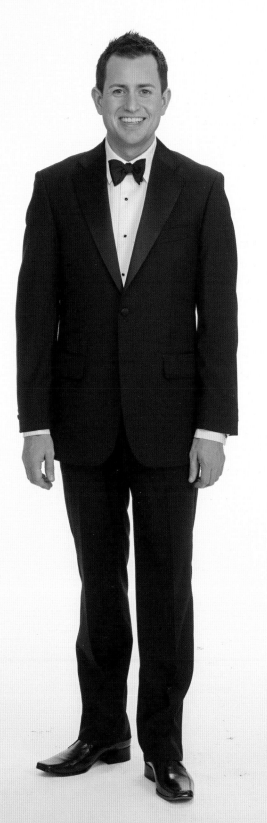

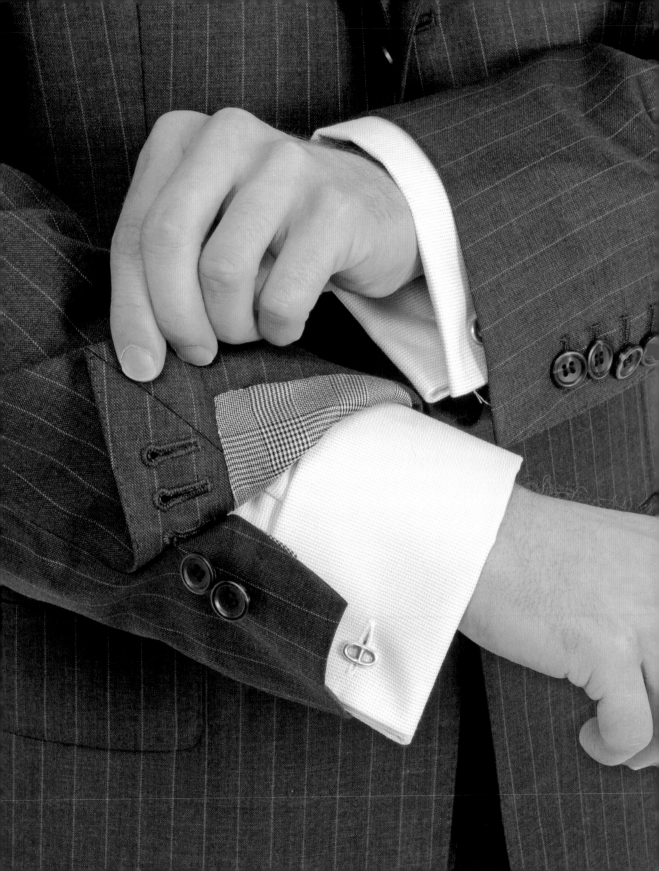

6

putting
it all
together

Suit tailoring

Buying a suit is a major investment (see pages 138–139), so selecting the right cut for your shape is essential. There are many variations when it comes to suits. Check the options below and the suit fabrics on pages 110–115 to ensure that you buy what is best for you.

The single-breasted jacket

The single-breasted jacket suits all body shapes and is the safest option if suits are not your everyday wear and a good business staple if you require a tailored wardrobe for work. You will find a wide choice of styles and fabrics, from the classic British with double vents to the American, with narrow lapels giving an elongating effect.

Button positioning

The positioning of the buttons on the jacket will depend on your proportions and on fashion:
One button approximately on your waistline.
Two buttons one above the waistline, one below.
Three buttons middle button on your waistline.
Jackets with more than three buttons are high-fashion looks and not necessarily an investment buy.

What to button?

If you are not sure which buttons to fasten, bear in mind the following:
Top button sometimes
Middle button always
Lower button never

If you're not sure what suits you, the single-breasted jacket is the safest option as it suits all body shapes.

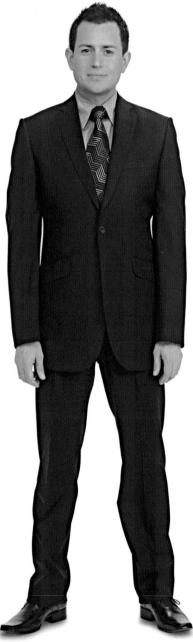

The double-breasted jacket

A double-breasted jacket is considered slightly more dressy than a single-breasted one.

Button positioning

The number of buttonholes does not always match the number of buttons on the double-breasted jacket.

Two buttons these are positioned side by side near the waistline.

Four buttons the positioning of the buttons will depend on the length of the jacket's collar – a short collar has two buttonholes, a long collar only one. The waist will be between the two rows of buttons.

Six buttons a jacket with a short collar has three buttonholes, a long collar only two.

What to button?

Always button the inside button when wearing the jacket closed. Whether there are two or three buttonholes, never button the bottom ones.

The choice is yours

Ready-made

A ready-made, or off-the-peg, suit is one that you buy from any store, normally sold as two separate pieces so that you can select the best ready-made size of jacket and trousers for you.

Made-to-measure

This is a pre-cut suit that will be adjusted and finished to your measurements. Your choice of lining and turn-ups (cuffs) are some of the options available to you on a made-to-measure suit.

Bespoke

A bespoke suit is cut and made up completely to your measurements, and often involves two fittings during making. You will have complete flexibility as to the design and finish of the suit.

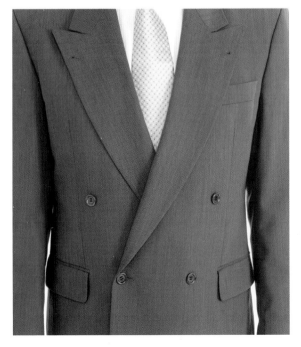

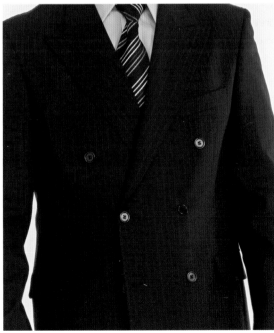

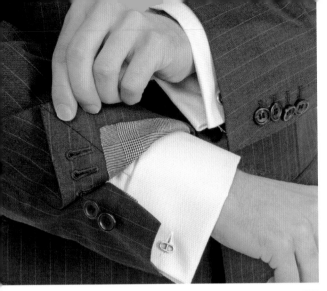

Jacket details

Cuffs

Historically, the lower two buttonholes on a sleeve cuff were always real so that the cuff could be rolled back and allow surgeons to operate without spoiling their clothes. These buttonholes are found today only on expensive designer-label suits and bespoke tailoring, though more young fashion brands are now adding these to their ready-to-wear lines to express quality.

Vents

Vents are the slits found along the bottom edge in the back of some jackets to allow for freedom of movement and easy access to the trouser pockets, without unsightly bunching or creasing of the jacket's line. There will either be a single vent in the middle, or two vents on either side of the back of the jacket. The choice between single and double vents really depends on the shape of your bottom. If you have curves there, double vents sit better.

Ventless jackets hug the hips. Be aware though that reaching into your trouser pockets or sitting will break the line of the jacket by bunching up around the waistline.

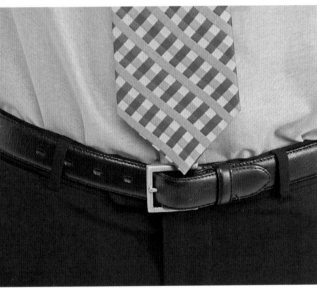

Trousers

Again, consider your body shape before deciding on the style of suit trousers to wear:
Flat-fronted should be avoided if you are Rounded.
Single-pleated suits all men.
Double-pleated suits most men.

Consider the following tips for wearing trousers:
Loops on waistband you must wear a suitable belt.
Braces (suspenders) these should preferably be buttoned only, not clipped.
Waist adjustments these are great if you have a tendency to a fluctuating waistline.
Turn-ups (cuffs) these depend on the styling of your suit, and are best avoided if you have short legs.

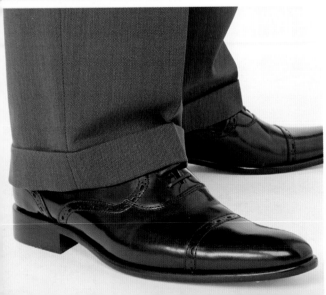

The British suit

British tailoring is the benchmark for men's tailoring worldwide, and follows traditions that go back many decades. The British-cut suit is the most constructed suit that you will find. An off-the-peg suit will have details that reflect the British-cut style, for example the close contouring of the jacket, the four buttons on the sleeves and the double vents.

Jacket characteristics

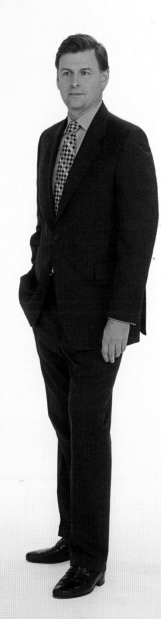

✓ It has a straight shoulder line, which is padded.

✓ The collar is notched with a buttonhole on the left-hand side.

✓ There is shaped waist definition.

✓ If single-breasted, the jacket has slightly curved front panels.

✓ If double-breasted, the jacket has straight front panels and broader lapels.

✓ It has a breast pocket on the left-hand side.

✓ There are flaps on the pockets.

Trousers have...

✓ A flat front

✓ Slashed pockets

✓ A ticket pocket

✓ Straight legs

✗ Traditionally no turn-ups (cuffs)

Fabric

The British-cut suit suits all type of fabrics from the lightest gabardines to heavyweight tweeds.

The Italian suit

The stylish Italian-cut suit is a more relaxed style of tailoring and is more fashionable than the traditional British cut. Its elegance is often reflected in the use of lightweight soft fabrics, combined with a greater selection of colours and patterns. It demonstrates the wearer's sense of, and appreciation of, fashion.

Jacket characteristics

✓ It has a slightly softer shoulder line, which extends beyond the natural shoulder line.

✓ The lapels are peaked and wider than the British-cut suit.

✓ The jacket hangs straight at the back, tapering into the bottom.

✓ At the back of the jacket there are slight folds at the sleeve edge.

✓ It has wider sleeves than a British cut.

✓ It has a breast pocket on the left-hand side.

The trousers have...

✓ Single or double pleats

✓ Slashed pockets

✓ A ticket pocket

✓ Full legs

Fabric

The Italian-cut suit suits luxurious cloths in light- or medium-weight wool.

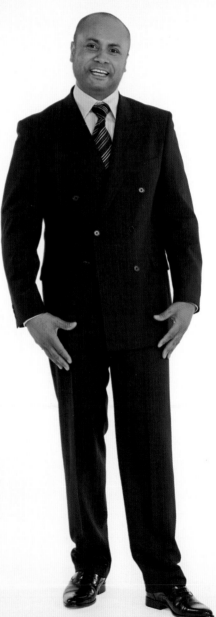

The American suit

The American-cut suit, also known as the sack suit, is the most relaxed form of tailoring. The first mass-produced suit, it allowed jackets and trousers to be sold separately. This made it possible to buy trousers with different waist measurements and leg lengths. The American suit is single-breasted only with, a single centre vent.

Jacket characteristics

✓ It has a soft rounded shoulder line.

✓ The lapels are notched but long.

✓ It is single-breasted with one or two buttons.

✓ It hangs straight.

✓ There is a breast pocket on the left-hand side.

✓ There are flap or patched pockets.

The trousers have...

✓ Single or double pleats

✓ Slashed pockets

✓ A ticket pocket

✓ Full legs

✓ Turn-ups (cuffs) or no turn-ups (cuffs)

Fabric

The American suit doesn't work in a fine crisp gabardine or worsted wool, but it is an excellent cut for linen, silk and wool/polyester mix.

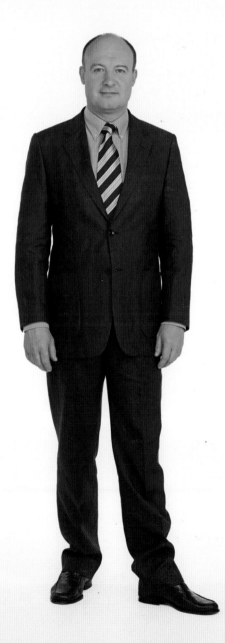

Suit fabrics for the **Light** Man

It is better for a man with light colouring to shop in the spring and summertime when lighter colours will be more easily available. Remember when wearing the darker shades of your palette to keep your shirt colours light; you will also need to consider the size of the pattern and the weight of the fabric so as to complement your scale and height.

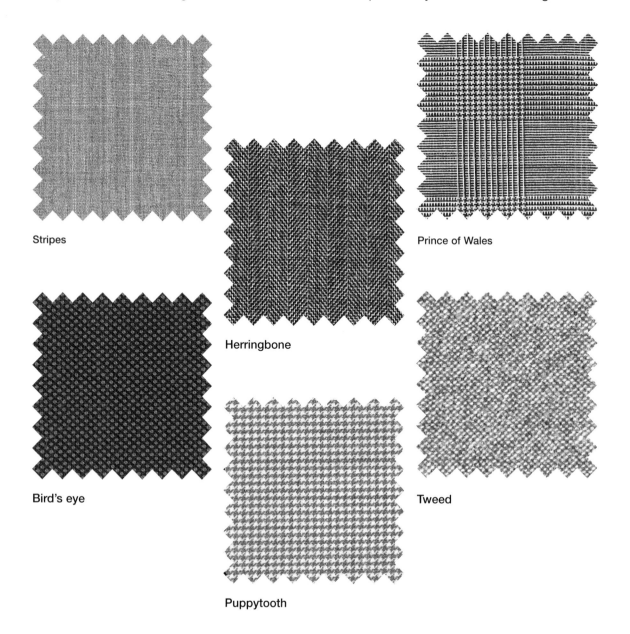

Stripes

Herringbone

Prince of Wales

Bird's eye

Puppytooth

Tweed

Suit fabrics for the **Deep** Man

Most of your suit fabrics will be available in the shops all year round. In the summertime choose a lightweight cool wool but keep within your darker colour palette. When choosing your stripe, consider your scale: a fine bone structure will look better in a narrow stripe, whilst a grand scale man will be complemented with a wider stripe.

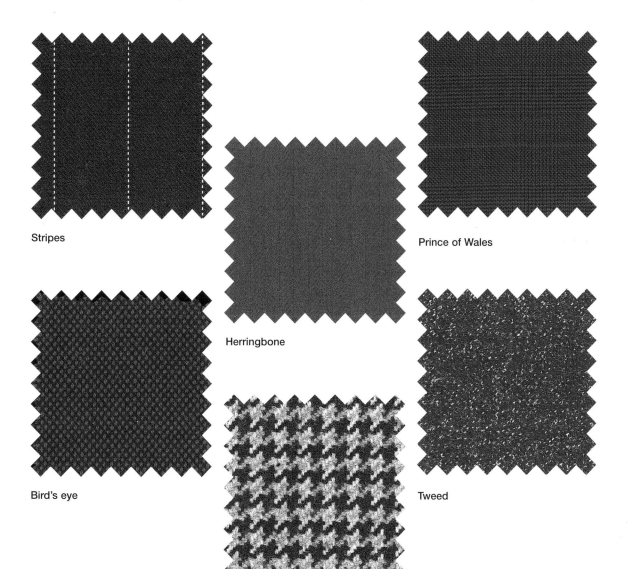

Stripes

Prince of Wales

Herringbone

Bird's eye

Tweed

Houndstooth

Suit fabrics for the **Warm** Man

The challenge for a man with warm colouring will be to abandon greys and navies. If this is not appropriate for your business environment, warm these up with cream and yellow shirts, making sure that your ties reflect the warm colours from your palette. A mint or light periwinkle shirt would look perfect with any of the suit fabrics below.

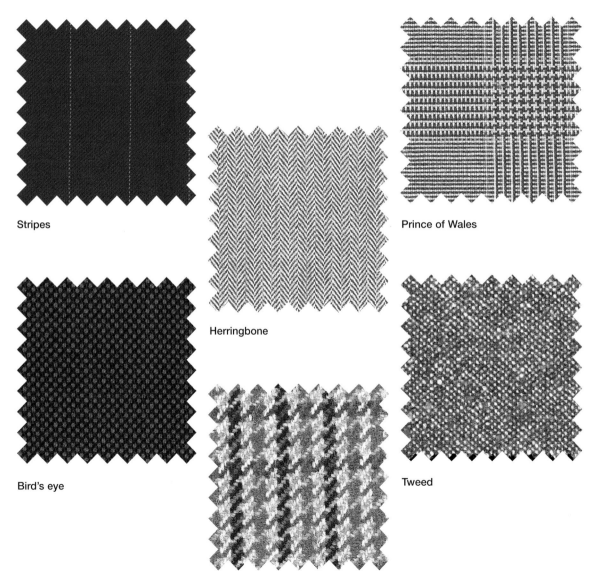

Stripes

Herringbone

Prince of Wales

Bird's eye

Houndstooth

Tweed

Suit fabrics for the **Cool** Man

Grey and and navy suit fabrics are ideal for the cool man, so you will have the widest choice of fabrics. If you have white hair and pale blue eyes, be careful not to go too dark with your navies. The best choice of shirt colours will be pinks, lavenders and blues. Include aquas and turquoise in your ties.

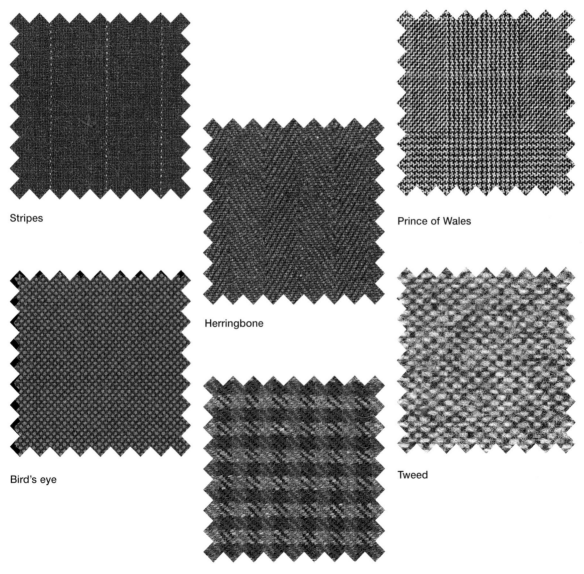

Stripes

Herringbone

Prince of Wales

Bird's eye

Houndstooth

Tweed

Suit fabrics for the **Clear** Man

The best look for the clear man is to opt for a cloth where the patterns are distinct and sharp. For example, the pinstripe and the black and white in the puppytooth below are sharp and distinctive in their contrast. If you choose to wear the bird's eye or tweed, you will need to ensure that your shirt and tie are bright and contrasting.

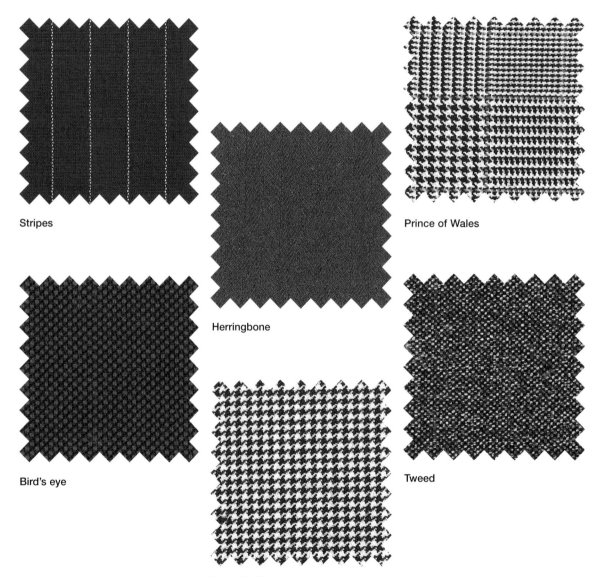

Stripes

Prince of Wales

Herringbone

Bird's eye

Puppytooth

Tweed

Suit fabrics for the **Muted** Man

A muted man should go for a tonal look so that colours blend in rather than contrast. You should opt for colours that are similar in tone and depth – they should be neither too dark nor too light. The colour of the stripe should also be muted and tonal. A soft white shirt will always look better on you than a pure white one.

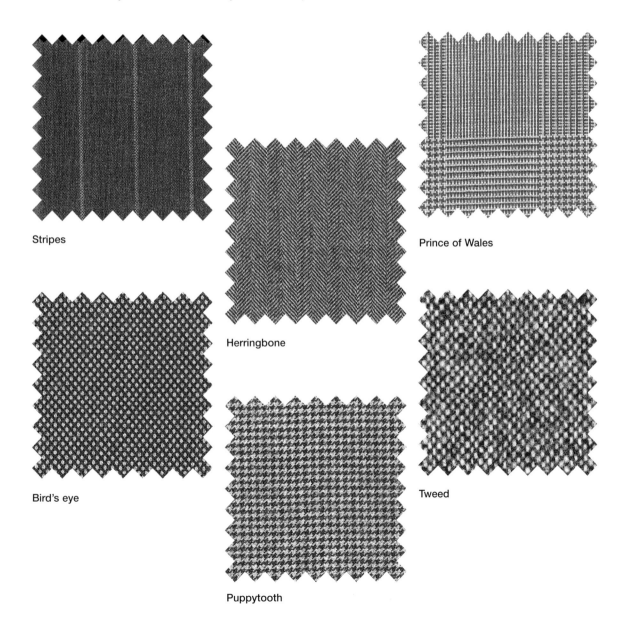

Stripes

Herringbone

Prince of Wales

Bird's eye

Puppytooth

Tweed

Making sure it fits

As a suit is an investment buy (see pages 138–139), it is important to get it right. Often the sales assistant is more interested in the sale than the fit, so it is down to you to know what to look for and what is a good fit and what is not. Take time over your choice and wear the appropriate clothing.

Jacket

✓ When buttoned there should be no bunching or wrinkling across the back and no tension lines pulling across the shoulder blades.

✓ There should be a slight vertical fold from the shoulder to allow for ease of movement. This is more exaggerated in an Italian-cut suit (see page 108).

✓ There should be enough movement in the jacket so that when it is buttoned it lies flat across the front of the chest or stomach for those who are slightly rounded. If you see an X formation around the button near the waist, then the jacket is too tight.

✓ The lapels of the jacket should lie flat across your chest; if they don't, the jacket is too small or the fabric is wrong for your body shape.

✓ When worn open, the jacket should hang straight down at the back and at the front, otherwise the balance of the suit is wrong.

✓ Beware that wide lapels and a wide shoulder line will make your head seem smaller, as indeed too narrow a lapel and a tight shoulder line will make your head look bigger.

✓ The jacket is the right length when it finishes just below the point where your bottom starts to curve under.

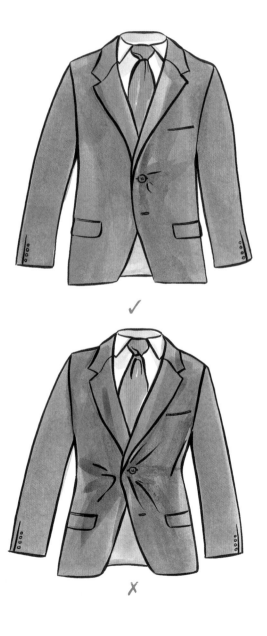

✓

✗

Collar

✓ The jacket needs to sit next to the shirt collar with no gap in between.

✓ The jacket collar should allow for at least 1.5 cm (¾ in) of the shirt collar to show.

✓ The collar must lie flat around your neck and not gape.

✓ You can have your collar adjusted by a tailor if it doesn't fit properly.

✓ Do not forget to balance the size of your tie knot (see pages 122–123) with that of your jacket lapel and shirt collar.

✓ To balance your look, choose the right shirt collar shape (see page 69).

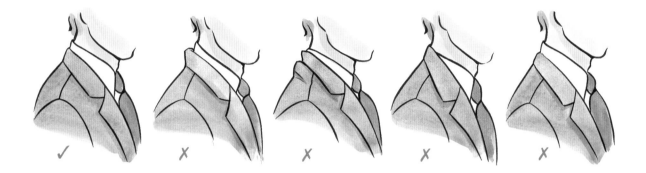

Sleeves

✓ The sleeve should finish where the wrist breaks with the hand and where the edge of the sleeve can rest on the back of the hand.

✓ There should always be at least 1.5 cm (¾ in) of shirt sleeve showing from under the jacket sleeves. However, if you have short arms, you will need to allow for 1 cm (½ in) only to peep out.

✓ Short-sleeved shirts should never be worn with a formal suit.

✓ The jacket sleeve should hang straight with no horizontal breaks on the upper arm and should narrow slightly towards the wrist.

✓ The bottom opening of the sleeve should measure approximately 15 cm (6 in) in diameter.

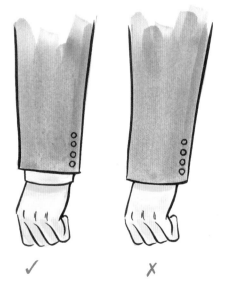

Shirt

✓ When your shirt collar is buttoned up, you should be able to place a finger between your neck and the shirt.

✓ Ensure that the shirt is long enough to tuck easily into your trousers so that when you lift your arms, the shirt tail does not come out.

✓ Different-length sleeves are available for those with extra long arms.

✓ The buttons on the front of the shirt should lie flat. Refer to your body shape (see pages 52–63) to ensure you choose the right-fitting shirt for you.

✓ If your shirt is too loose and baggy, try buying one in a different weight of cotton – a fine, crisp fabric will hold its shape better.

Tips

• When shopping for a new suit or a jacket/trousers combination wear the type of shirt and tie you would normally wear, together with the correct shoes and socks. You cannot judge the fit correctly if you are wearing a t-shirt and trainers.

• Don't overload either your jacket or trouser pockets with boy toys: mobile phone, blackberry, Ipod, keys or a bulky wallet. All of these will spoil the sleek lines of your clothes.

• It is important to try on a shirt before you buy it, as every designer-label or store brand will size their shirts differently.

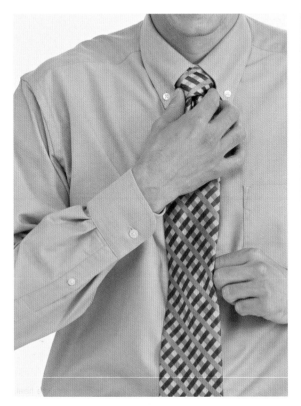
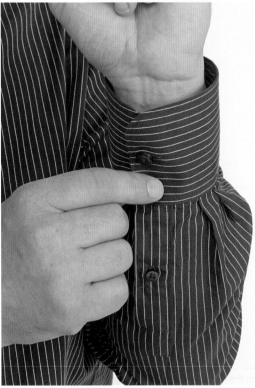

Trousers

✓ The waistband of your trousers should be worn as near to your natural waistline as possible. If trousers are worn under the fuller stomach this means the crotch hangs low and the leg length is incorrect.

✓ The waistband should lie flat at the waist, and not curl over (a sign that the waist of the trousers is too small).

✓ If the trouser legs have creases these should be maintained at all times and should run down the centre of the legs and fall in the middle of your shoes. If the trouser leg twists around, you may need to consider a different style or wider-legged trousers.

✓ If the trousers have turn-ups (cuffs) they should fall with one break across the shoe. If they don't have turn-ups (cuffs) they should have one break but can also slant back slightly over the heel on the shoe. Your socks should not be visible.

✓ If the trousers have belt loops, a belt is a must. A bespoke suit does not have belt loops as the trousers will have been made to fit exactly and may have an adjustment strap on the side.

✓ Straight or slanted side pockets should lie flat and not gape (an indication that the trousers are too tight).

✓ Fashion often determines whether there are pleats in trousers (Italian-cut suit) or not (British cut). Men with a fuller stomach will find that the pleats provide extra comfort and movement.

✓ The length of your trousers should be sufficient to rest on the top of your shoe and to conceal your socks when in full stride and cover any flesh when seated. Some narrow cut trousers may sit higher.

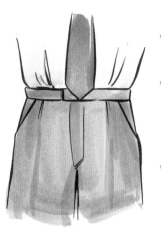

Trousers should be worn on the waist.

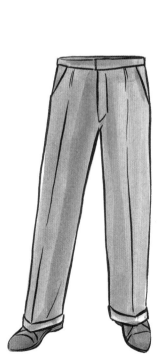

Trouser creases should centre on the knee and shoe.

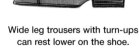

Wide leg trousers with turn-ups can rest lower on the shoe.

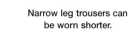

Narrow leg trousers can be worn shorter.

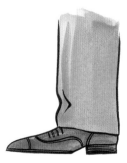

Trousers with no turn-ups should slant towards the heel.

Combining suits, ties and shirts

The chart below provides stylish suit, shirt and tie combinations, whatever the occasion. The important rules to remember are that when combining just two patterns, the colours must be complementary. When combining three patterns, the colours must be the same, and the patterns must be of the same design although not the same size.

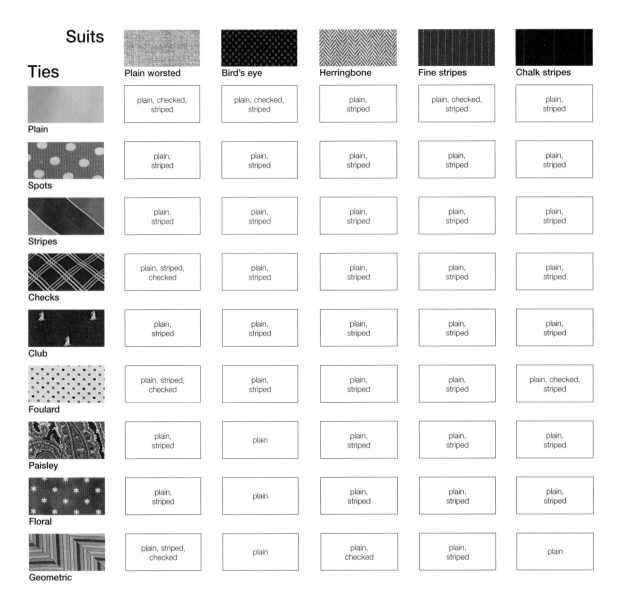

Ties \ Suits	Plain worsted	Bird's eye	Herringbone	Fine stripes	Chalk stripes
Plain	plain, checked, striped	plain, checked, striped	plain, striped	plain, checked, striped	plain, striped
Spots	plain, striped	plain, striped	plain, striped	plain, striped	plain, striped
Stripes	plain, striped	plain, striped	plain, striped	plain, striped	plain, striped
Checks	plain, striped, checked	plain, striped	plain, striped	plain, striped	plain, striped
Club	plain, striped	plain, striped	plain, striped	plain, striped	plain, striped
Foulard	plain, striped, checked	plain, striped	plain, striped	plain, striped	plain, checked, striped
Paisley	plain, striped	plain	plain, striped	plain, striped	plain, striped
Floral	plain, striped	plain	plain, striped	plain, striped	plain, striped
Geometric	plain, striped, checked	plain	plain, checked	plain, striped	plain

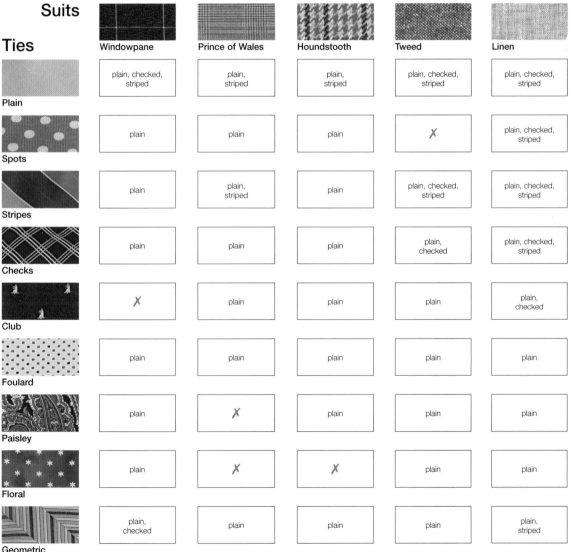

	Suits				
Ties	**Windowpane**	**Prince of Wales**	**Houndstooth**	**Tweed**	**Linen**
Plain	plain, checked, striped	plain, striped	plain, striped	plain, checked, striped	plain, checked, striped
Spots	plain	plain	plain	✗	plain, checked, striped
Stripes	plain	plain, striped	plain	plain, checked, striped	plain, checked, striped
Checks	plain	plain	plain	plain, checked	plain, checked, striped
Club	✗	plain	plain	plain	plain, checked
Foulard	plain	plain	plain	plain	plain
Paisley	plain	✗	plain	plain	plain
Floral	plain	✗	✗	plain	plain
Geometric	plain, checked	plain	plain	plain	plain, striped

How to tie ties

The tie is your most important formal wear accessory and gives you the opportunity to use colour with flair and a little restraint – you need to be remembered afterwards, not your tie! Whatever the colour or pattern of your tie, the way you tie it must be right for your scale and proportions. See pages 68–69 to find out which tie knot is best for you.

Tying a school boy tie

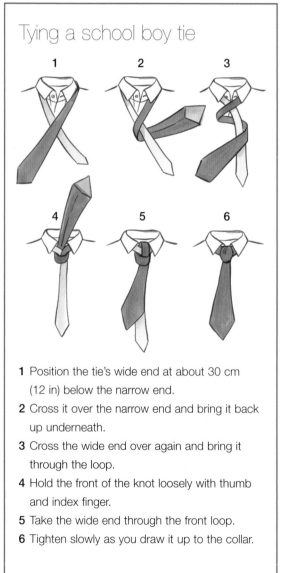

1 Position the tie's wide end at about 30 cm (12 in) below the narrow end.
2 Cross it over the narrow end and bring it back up underneath.
3 Cross the wide end over again and bring it through the loop.
4 Hold the front of the knot loosely with thumb and index finger.
5 Take the wide end through the front loop.
6 Tighten slowly as you draw it up to the collar.

Tying a half Windsor

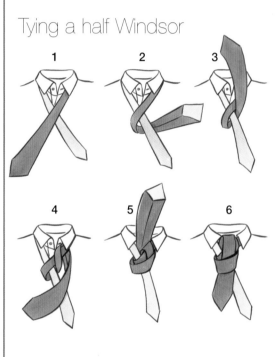

1 Position the tie's wide end at about 30 cm (12 in) below the narrow end.
2 Cross it over the narrow end and bring it back underneath.
3 Take the wide end up through the loop.
4 Pass it around the front from left to right.
5 Bring it through the loop again and pass it through the knot in front.
6 Tighten slowly as you draw it up to the collar.

Tie Tips

- The knot of your tie must fit close to the collar of your shirt so that no gap is visible between them.
- The tip of your tie should rest just above the waistband or belt on your trousers. The tail of the tie should not be seen.

Tying a double Windsor

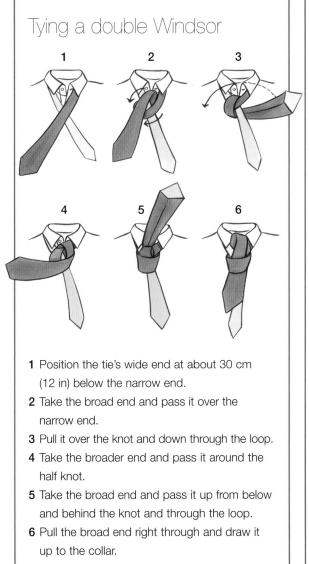

1 Position the tie's wide end at about 30 cm (12 in) below the narrow end.
2 Take the broad end and pass it over the narrow end.
3 Pull it over the knot and down through the loop.
4 Take the broader end and pass it around the half knot.
5 Take the broad end and pass it up from below and behind the knot and through the loop.
6 Pull the broad end right through and draw it up to the collar.

Tying a bow tie

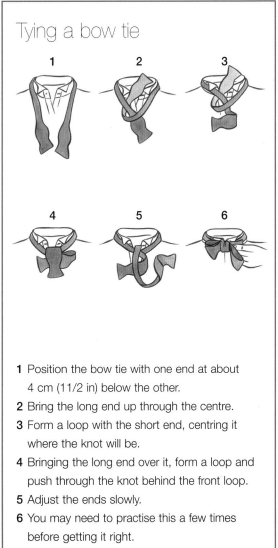

1 Position the bow tie with one end at about 4 cm (11/2 in) below the other.
2 Bring the long end up through the centre.
3 Form a loop with the short end, centring it where the knot will be.
4 Bringing the long end over it, form a loop and push through the knot behind the front loop.
5 Adjust the ends slowly.
6 You may need to practise this a few times before getting it right.

Shoes

The shoes you wear should depend on the clothes you are wearing. To maintain the image of the well-dressed man your shoes need to complete your look. The wrong shoes can completely destroy the effort you have put into choosing an outfit. Do not forget that the colour you select will also affect the whole look.

What to wear when

For formal or business wear leather shoes are a must. Balance the look of a formal British suit with lace-ups or buckled shoes. With an Italian or an American suit a more relaxed style might be more appropriate, such as some form of loafers or lightweight lace-ups.

When it comes to casual wear try to match your shoes to the style of your trousers. For example chinos and jeans go well with boat shoes or desert boots. If you like to wear cropped cargos or shorts, Birkenstocks or flip-flops (thongs) look best. Never wear socks with sandals.

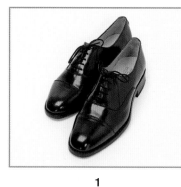

1

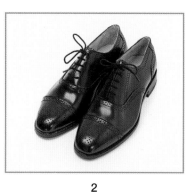

2

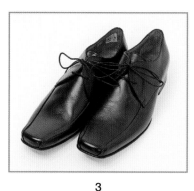

3

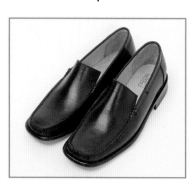

4

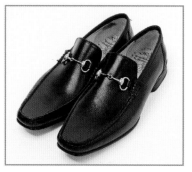

5

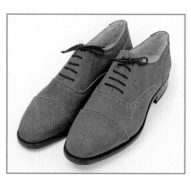

6

Getting the right size of shoes will ensure comfort and avoid long-term damage to your feet. Certain styles will be more comfortable for certain shape feet. Lace-up/adjustable fittings will be the most comfortable for someone with a high instep. Leather will be the most comfortable if you stand all day. Do adjust the weight of socks to the style/weight of the shoes: the heavier the shoes, the heavier the socks should be. Avoid wearing the same shoes two days in a row to give them a chance to 'breathe'. It will be easier to clean your shoes as soon as you remove them as the warmth will make them softer.

Formal shoes

1 Oxford plains
2 Oxford brogues
3 Plain lace-ups
4 Plain loafers
5 Buckled loafers
6 Brown suede lace-ups (leather sole)

Casual shoes

7 Birkenstock-type
8 Desert boot
9 Trainers
10 Canvas shoes
11 Boat shoes
12 High-fashion trainers

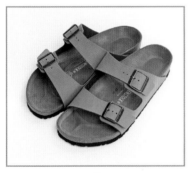

7

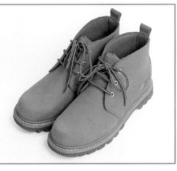

8

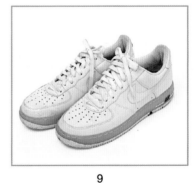

9

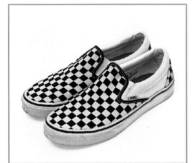

10

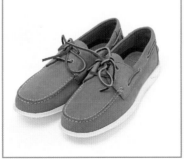

11

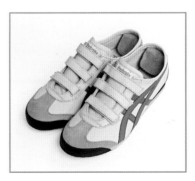

12

Underwear

It's important to consider what clothes you'll be wearing before deciding what underwear to select for that day. Change all items of underwear every day, and even twice a day in a hot climate or after any form of exercise. The style of underwear you choose is down to personal choice and the degree of comfort that is required.

Vests (undershirts)

Wearing a vest (undershirt) is dictated by culture, preferences, weather conditions and sensitivity to fabrics. Traditionally, vests (undershirts) were worn as an extra layer to add warmth and to protect the shirt from soiling. Vests (undershirts) are now worn for warmth but also to absorb perspiration in hot conditions.

If you do choose to wear a vest (undershirt) or t-shirt, you must ensure that it does not show through the outer garment, especially if you are wearing a formal shirt.

Vest (undershirt) The standard vest (undershirt) comes in different versions – from a plain cotton interlock to a string vest (undershirt). A vest (undershirt) of this type is never worn on its own, however hot it is!

Thermal vest (undershirt) A long- or short-sleeved thermal vest (undershirt) will help keep you warm in cold weather conditions. Thermal comes in various fabrics including wool and silk for extra warmth; make sure it is suitable for the purpose.

Under t-shirt If you choose to wear a t-shirt beneath your shirt, make sure it is a lightweight one that does not show through the top fabric, although the neckline may be seen on an open-necked shirt.

Underpants (shorts)

Again, this is a question of personal choice and once a man has found his favourite style he is unlikely to change it. In the last 20 years, however, many new designs have become available due to fabric technology developments and fashion trends. For maximum comfort, cotton is always best. Do make sure that no underwear is visible above the waistline of your trousers, and that there is no visible pant line (VPL) showing through the trouser fabric.

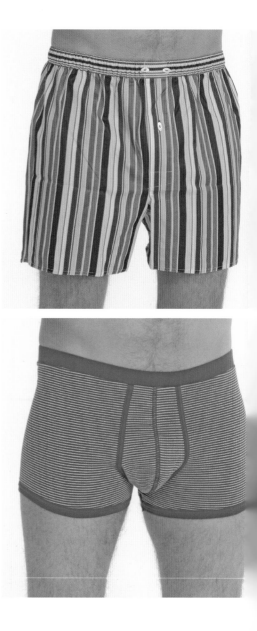

Briefs (jockey shorts) These are good for wearing under tight or close-fitting trousers, with low-rise trousers and under sportswear.

Y- or A-fronts A traditional men's underpants (shorts), which can be worn under most garments.

Trunks Made popular by Calvin Klein, this is now the norm for men's underpants (shorts). The cotton/Lycra mix offers good support.

Boxer shorts Generally made of 100 per cent cotton with an elasticated and gathered waistband, boxers are ideal underwear for sensitive skin or in hot weather conditions.

Socks

You need a wardrobe of socks to give you a choice for different occasions. When sock shopping, always buy at least three pairs of each type to beat the 'washing machine gobbler' and buy them in a size larger than you need as they will shrink. Although they may appear to be a small item, socks are a key accessory that says a lot about your style and dress sense. For understated style, the colour of your socks should coordinate with your trousers. Character socks given to you as a present do not have to be worn all the time!

Formal business wear Choose long socks in either a wool or cotton mix in plain, dark neutral colours.

Business casual wear Go for long or three-quarter length socks, in plain colours in either a wool or cotton mix. Remember to coordinate the colour of your socks with that of your trousers.

Smart casual Wear three-quarter length argyle-type socks, or subtle patterns. The colours should tone with your trousers.

Casual This is when you can wear your character socks.

Sportswear Sports shoes, for example for golfing, football, tennis or cycling, normally have a specified type of sock. Wear either trainers socks or white sports socks with trainers, and heavyweight wool or cotton mix with walking boots.

Evening dress Long black silk socks are the socks of choice.

Sockless Leave off the socks with open sandals. You can choose to go sockless with leather boat shoes in a hot climate, and with lightweight leather loafers for a smart casual look. Do not be tempted to go sockless with trainers if you want to keep your friends!

Colour clashing socks As a fashion statement you may choose to wear, say, red socks with a suit. This can work for a business casual look if you are a Creative, Dramatic or Romantic (see pages 76–81).

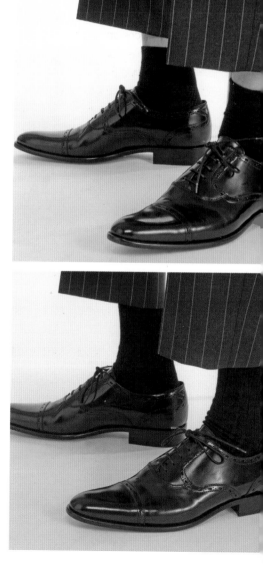

Revealing your calves is not a good look – long socks will make sure that this doesn't happen.

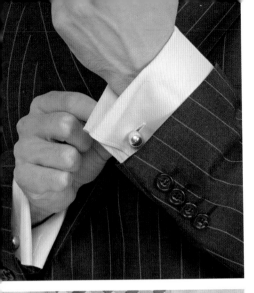

Choosing accessories

Accessories – from a handkerchief to a bag – are a great opportunity to express a little individuality and it can be fun to shop for them yourself, following your signature style and colour guidelines. Select items that will be appropriate to the rest of your outfit – keeping smart and casual separate where necessary.

The accessories you choose to wear depend a lot on your personal look and preferences. Getting it right is also what makes you that well-dressed man.

Cufflinks

Cufflinks are worn only with shirts with a double (French) cuff. Make sure they are appropriate for the occasion. Silk knots are a cheap but colourful way to dress a formal shirt.

Belts

Always wear one if your trousers or shorts have belt loops. The belt needs to complement the outfit – for formal trousers choose a fine leather belt with a simple buckle, for casual trousers or jeans opt for a heavier weight belt and buckle.

Braces (suspenders)

These are often worn with formal wear and the classic buttoned version is preferable. Clip-on braces are more readily available but shouldn't be worn if belt loops are visible.

Handkerchiefs

Always carry a clean cotton handkerchief with you. Silk handkerchiefs can add a dash of colour to an otherwise dark formal suit or sports jacket, if you feel this is your style. It should be in a complementary colour but never the same pattern as your tie.

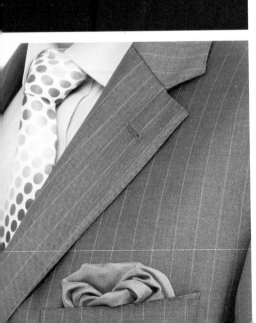

Watches

Your watch should balance with your scale and proportions (see pages 64–67). You should also consider having a selection of watches for different occasions – a sports watch for beachwear, for example, is not appropriate with a dinner suit.

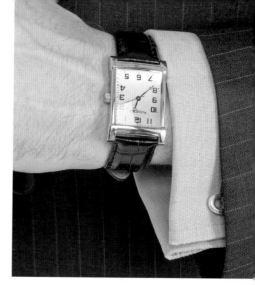

Jewellery

Rings For most men, a ring will simply be a wedding ring, signet or graduation ring. The more creative among you may wish to wear other rings; just make sure that they are appropriate for the occasion.
Necklaces Unless you wear a necklace with a religious symbol, wearing necklaces is appropriate only with casual wear.
Earrings Check with your employers on their dress code to see whether wearing earrings, or indeed any other body piercing, is acceptable to them.

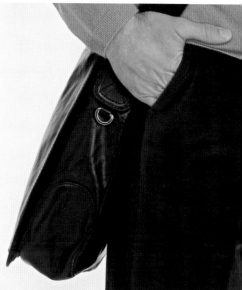

Bags

With so many gadgets to keep with you nowadays – iPods, laptops, mobile phones – in addition to your keys, wallet and any business papers, you may need to consider getting a bag. Carrying even small objects in your jacket or trouser pockets is not a solution.

The type of bag you choose depends on what it is required to hold and when and where you will be using it. Consider the weight of what you carry around, and see whether a back-pack or wheeled case would be more suitable.

Formal options
Briefcase
Attaché case
Flight case
Document case
Photographer's case

Casual options
Satchel (leather or canvas) or despatch bag
Back-pack
Hold-all

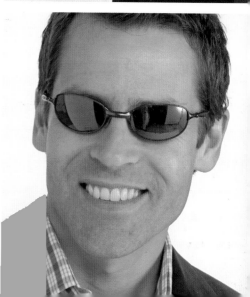

Core wardrobe

You don't need a vast wardrobe of clothes to be well dressed for work and formal occasions. The important thing is to rotate your clothes and shoes on a daily basis to allow your clothes to rest between wearing. The numbers of items quoted below are the minimum requirements to ensure you are well dressed at all times.

Formal wardrobe

3 suits (navy, charcoal, other dark neutral from your colour palette) or 3 jacket-and-trouser combinations
5 working shirts
5 silk ties in colours coordinating with your shirts
1 outer coat
2–3 pairs of shoes (Oxford brogues, Oxford plains and buckled shoes, see pages 124–125)
1 leather belt

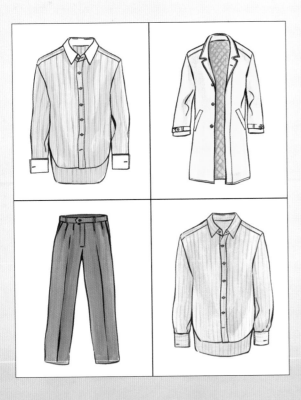

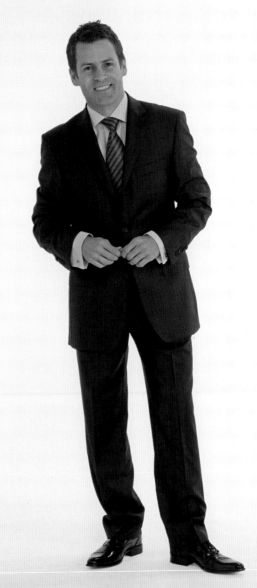

To make your core wardrobe work, rotate your clothes and shoes on a daily basis and ensure that shirts and suits, or trousers, coordinate within your colour palette.

Casual wardrobe

2 pairs of casual trousers
2 pairs of jeans
8 shirts or t-shirts
2 sweaters
1 casual jacket
2 pairs of appropriate shoes or boots (boat shoes,
Timberlands or high-fashion trainers, see page 125)
1 casual belt

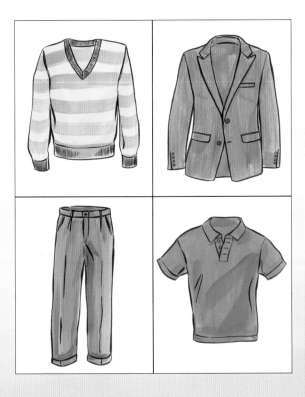

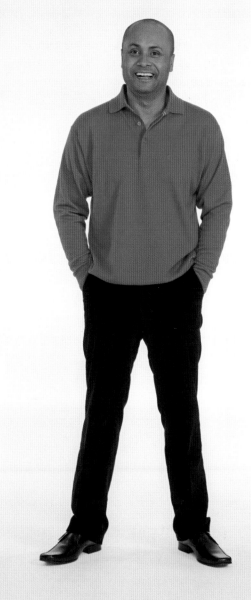

Looking after your clothes

To ensure you get the optimum length of wear from your clothes and the best return on your investment buys (see pages 138–139), you need a good routine for looking after them. This involves making sure they look clean, are well pressed and show no obvious signs of wear and tear.

Suits and jackets

✓ Dry clean your suits no more than three times a year, unless soiled. With its use of chemicals, dry cleaning prematurely ages clothes and can break down the fusing in a jacket, so that the jacket appears wrinkled.

✓ Always empty the pockets of your jacket, button it up, pull out any flaps and hang it on a shaped wooden hanger after wearing. Leave outside your wardrobe to breathe overnight or replace in your cupboard, ensuring the air can circulate around it.

✓ Steam bi-monthly by hanging in the bathroom while running a bath or shower.

✓ Allow two to three days between each wearing as your suit can absorb up to 600 ml (1 pint) of water during one wearing!

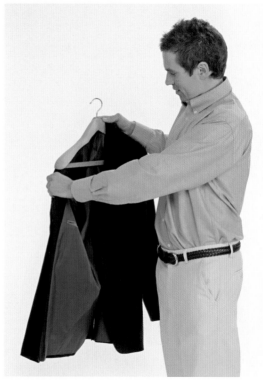

Non-washable trousers

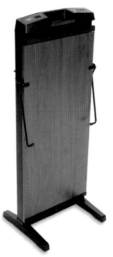

✓ After each wearing, empty the pockets and remove the belt.

✓ The simplest way of looking after your trousers is to invest in a trouser press.

✓ If possible always hang your trousers from the waist or the bottom. If you have to fold your trousers use a padded trouser hanger to avoid the tell-tale fold.

✓ Before putting any item back in the wardrobe, check for loose buttons and any wear on the bottom of your trousers.

Washable trousers and jeans

✓ Before laundering, read the care label as different fabrics need different care – some need tumble drying and others line drying.

✓ Empty the pockets and turn the trousers inside out before washing – this ensures the fabric fades less and is less prone to rub-fading.

✓ Don't leave trousers in the washing machine for too long when the cycle has finished, as they will crease even more.

Shirts

✓ Good quality cotton shirts don't need starching after washing.

✓ If you have the space, plastic-coated hangers are best for hanging shirts after laundering.

✓ Check collar and cuffs for fraying and replace any missing buttons.

Ties

✓ Avoid dry cleaning if you can as, ideally, ties should be unstitched and cleaned open, and restitched afterwards. Alternatively, remove any dirty spot with dry cleaning fluid on a white cotton cloth. Clean from the outside to the centre of the spot.

✓ When tying your tie knot, make sure your hands are absolutely clean to avoid tell-tale fingermarks on the knot.

✓ Undo the knot after every single wearing and hang the tie on a tie hanger.

✓ If crumpled, hang the tie in the bathroom while running a bath or shower to refresh it in the steam.

Sweaters

✓ Read the care label and follow the instructions.

✓ Only put away sweaters that are clean, and fold them neatly before replacing in the wardrobe.

✓ Use mothballs or bags to protect your knitwear.

✓ Don't be tempted to store sweaters in polythene bags as this won't allow the fabric to breathe.

Shoes

✓ Polish shoes frequently, ideally when they are still warm from wear, so that the leather absorbs the polish more easily.

✓ Store shoes on a rack. Placing shoe trees in your shoes before putting them away will prevent curling toes and wrinkled uppers.

✓ Check the soles and heels regularly and have them repaired by a good cobbler before they become too worn.

✓ Canvas shoes and trainers can be washed in the washing machine.

✓ Check laces (shoestrings) regularly and keep spares. White and light-coloured laces (shoestrings) should be washed.

Packing your bags

Whether you are travelling away from home for work or for pleasure, a little forethought and planning will go a long way. The checklist of packing rules below will help you keep things simple and organized, and the packing planners will ensure that you don't forget any essential items.

Packing rules

✓ Take as little as possible on your trip.

✓ Wear your heaviest shoes. Pack socks and other small soft items in the shoes that you pack.

✓ Empty all pockets in the clothes that you pack.

✓ Buy travel-sized toiletries and keep them only for travelling – you can also collect small shampoos and shower gels from hotels. For long stays, purchase toiletries on arrival – your bags will be lighter and there is no risk of products leaking.

✓ Take a small waterproof bag for packing any wet/dirty clothes on your return journey.

✓ Go through the packing planners opposite.

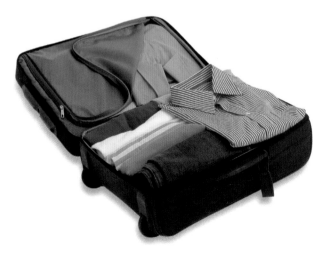

How to fold your clothes

To prevent creasing, the easiest way to pack clothes like jeans, t-shirts and casual shirts is to roll them.

Formal jackets

1 Hold the jacket facing you with your hands inside the shoulders.
2 Turn the left shoulder inside out.
3 Place the right shoulder inside the left – the lining is now facing outwards and the sleeves are folded inside.
4 Fold the jacket in half and lie it flat in your suitcase.

Formal shirts

1 Button every other button, starting with the top one.
2 Lie the shirt face down.
3 Fold a quarter of the way in across the yoke, bringing in the sleeves.
4 Fold one-third of the shirt from the tail up, and then fold again.
5 When packing shirts in the case, don't pile all the collars on top of each other.

Formal trousers

Fold them carefully along the crease, then fold in half. Lay pairs of trousers alternately in the suitcase so that not all the waistbands are together.

Shoes

Always pack shoes at the bottom of the case so that when the case is lifted they don't crush the clothes.

Packing planner: three-night business trip

Assuming that laundry facilities are not available you will need the following:

1 sports/casual jacket

1 pair of smart trousers

1 navy suit

1 grey suit

1 pair of jeans (note that
  you'll have no chance of

a flight upgrade if you
  wear these for travelling)

1 t-shirt

1 polo shirt

1 casual shirt

3 formal shirts

1 pair of formal shoes

1 pair of loafers

4 pairs of underpants
  (shorts)

5 pairs of socks

3 ties

2 belts

3 white handkerchiefs

Day	am/pm	Evening
1 – travel	Jacket, trousers, casual shirt, loafers	Change to polo shirt, keep loafers
2	Navy suit, formal shirt 1, tie 1, formal shoes	Change to jeans + t-shirt, loafers
3	Grey suit, formal shirt 2, tie 2, formal shoes	Grey suit, formal shirt 2, tie 3, formal shoes
Work + travel home	Navy suit, formal shirt 3, tie 1, formal shoes	

Packing planner: six-night beach holiday

Again, assuming that laundry facilities are not available you will need the items listed below. If laundry is available, you can cut your total of shirts/t-shirts and underwear by half.

1 casual jacket

1 pair of casual trousers

2 pairs of jeans

3 pairs of shorts (1 could
be a pair of cut-offs)

5 t-shirts

3 polo or casual shirts

1 pair of boat shoes

1 pair of sandals/flip-
flops (thongs)

1 pair of high-fashion
trainers

8 pairs of underpants
(shorts)

3 pairs of socks

1 belt

2 pairs of swimming
trunks

1 hat/cap

suntan lotion

Day	am/pm	Evening
1 – travel	Casual jacket, shirt 1, trousers, boat shoes	Jeans 1, shirt 2, boat shoes
2	Shorts 1, t-shirt 1, sandals/flip-flops (thongs)	Trousers, polo shirt 1, boat shoes
3	Shorts 2, t-shirt 2, sandals/flip-flops (thongs)	Jeans 2, polo shirt 2, trainers
4	Shorts 3, t-shirt 3, sandals/flip-flops (thongs)	Jeans 1, t-shirt 4, trainers
5	Shorts 1, t-shirt 4, sandals/flip-flops (thongs)	Jeans 2, t-shirt 5, trainers
6	Shorts 2, t-shirt 5, sandals/flip-flops (thongs)	Shorts 3, polo shirt 3, boat shoes
Travel home	Casual jacket, shirt 2, trousers, boat shoes	

Auditing your wardrobe

Before looking at the contents of your wardrobe and making a plan for your clothing needs, first ensure that your clothes are working efficiently for you. Give yourself enough time to examine them all and then eliminate from your wardrobe any items that don't work for you.

Audit your clothes

Go through all your clothes, one by one, and ask yourself the following questions about each one:

✓ Does it still fit?

✓ Is it in good condition?

✓ Is it the right colour?

✓ Is it the right style?

✓ Do I still have a use for it with my present lifestyle?

✓ Is it current?

If the answer to any of the above questions is 'No', take that particular garment to the charity shop.

If you haven't worn something for over 18 months, ask yourself why you are keeping it. Don't hoard just for the sake of it.

Assessing and planning

By analysing your lifestyle and how you spend your time, you will be able to assess whether your current wardrobe is suitable. To help you, create two pie charts. Divide the first chart into sections reflecting how you divide your day, and the second into sections which represent the contents of your wardrobe.

The pie charts should match one another. If they don't, you need to put together a shopping plan to address the shortfalls.

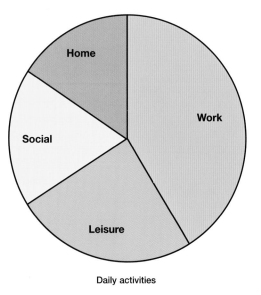

Daily activities

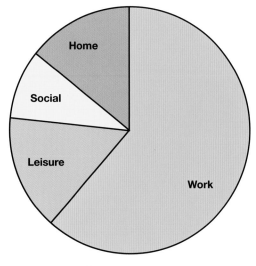

Contents of wardrobe

Wardrobe checklist

Refer to the core wardrobe on pages 130–131 for the basic number of pieces you need in your wardrobe. What you need to buy will depend on your lifestyle and what you already possess that is still relevant to your situation.

	Clothes I have	Clothes I need
Suits		
Formal jackets		
Formal trousers		
Formal shirts		
Ties		
Formal belts		
Formal socks		
Formal shoes		
Smart overcoat		
Evening wear		
Casual jackets		
Casual trousers		
Jeans		
Shorts		
Casual belts		
Casual/polo shirts		
T-shirts		
Sweaters		
Waterproof jackets		
Casual shoes		
Vests (undershirts)		
Underpants (shorts)		
Casual socks		

Shopping made easy

Once you have established what needs to be eliminated from your wardrobe and what you need to buy, make a shopping list and set yourself a budget. Remember to spend the most on what you wear the most. If a business suit is your work uniform, make it an investment buy; if jeans are your chosen work wear, make sure they fit you well.

Investment versus fashion buying

When it comes to buying clothes it is worth spending more than usual on something like a suit, a coat, waxed jacket or other outerwear, which you might buy only every few years. These are so-called investment buys. Shoes are often considered an investment buy, particularly if your lifestyle requires you to wear formal leather shoes. Remember that quality items will last longer than cheaper pieces, but you need to look after them (see pages 132–133) to ensure they last their anticipated lifetime.

As for fashion buys, your style personality (see Chapter 4) will determine whether you go for these or not. Fashion buys should be reserved for items that are less costly and that you won't mind not wearing in a year's time. Whether it is a shirt, a scarf, a sweater or shoes, a fashion buy lets you have fun adding style and colour to your investment wardrobe. Although you may not be into fashion, remember that staying current shows that you care about your image and how you project yourself. Of course, if you are into fashion and designer labels, fashion shopping is a lifestyle for you!

Do your research

It's worthwhile spending a little time researching where best to shop for your requirements and budget. Nothing is more frustrating than trailing around a shopping mall and not finding what you are after. A little forethought can guarantee your shopping trip is a happy and successful one.

✓ Check the internet for prices and store location.

✓ Read men's fashion magazines or the men's fashion columns in newspapers to keep abreast of what is current.

✓ Ask well-dressed friends and colleagues where they shop.

✓ Seek advice from an image consultant.

✓ Select stores where you know you will be offered expert advice.

✓ Avoid, if possible, shopping at the weekends when the staff may not have the time to look after you.

Dress for clothes shopping

Don't go shopping looking scruffy. You won't get the service you deserve, and the image reflecting back at you will not be the most positive. In addition, depending on what you are shopping for, you need to dress accordingly. If shopping for a suit, you need to wear a formal shirt and tie, together with the correct formal shoes. For casual wear, you need to wear the appropriate shoes. Don't wear too many layers when clothes shopping, as it will only mean more to take on and off when trying on clothes.

Where to shop

There are a multitude of options when it comes to *where* to buy your clothes – from department stores and specialist men's stores to catalogue and internet shopping. Choose the one that is right for you, with the environment in which you feel comfortable.

If going shopping in person, take with you someone whom you know will give you an honest opinion. (See pages 116–117 for ensuring a proper fit.)

Department stores

You will get the largest selection of styles and prices here and you will be able to browse without the interference of any overattentive sales people. When you want a sales assistant's help look for one who is well dressed and groomed.

Specialist men's stores

Specializing only in men's clothes, these shops include all prices from economy ranges to those offering bespoke tailoring. You may not feel quite so at ease to browse and wander around, but you are likely to find helpful staff. Choose a store that suits your lifestyle and budget and you'll be able to return time and time again, and the staff will get to know you and your taste.

Measure yourself

You need to know what size you are before buying clothes. Some department stores and all specialist men's stores have the facilities to measure you. You'll need to find out the following measurements:

Collar
Chest
Sleeve length – this is measured from the middle of your back across the shoulder and down your arm to just above the wrist.
Waist
Inside leg
Shoe size – this will also tell you what size socks to buy. Always buy your socks a size bigger than you think you need to allow for shrinkage in the wash.

Supermarkets

These are a great place to shop if you are on a limited budget and like to buy lots of fashionable items. They are ideal for sportswear and holiday wear.

Catalogue and internet shopping

If you hate shopping this may be the answer as you can browse at your leisure in the comfort of your own home. A catalogue often shows you how pieces work together for an overall look, which takes away the guesswork. Also, when the goods reach you, you can try them with items of clothing you already have in your wardrobe.

Do make sure that you keep all records of what you buy and return so as to make sure that you are not overcharged.

Who can wear what

When you next go shopping, make sure you have in mind all that you have learnt in this book. The following pages show the different styles within each general clothing category, some will be more suited to your personal style than others. Consider body shape, scale, proportions, colour and when you're going to wear it.

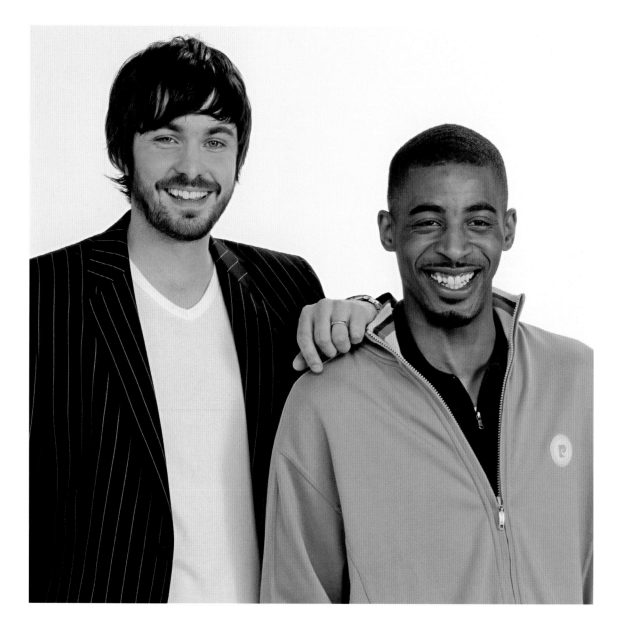

Shirts

All body shapes can wear all styles of shirts. Considerations are: fabrics, patterns and the shape of the collar.

1 Soft collar casual.
2 Short sleeve.
3 Granddad (not for a short neck).
4 Button-down Oxford.
5 Single cuff.
6 Double cuff.

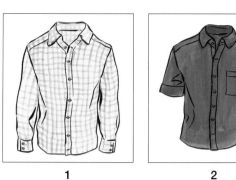

1

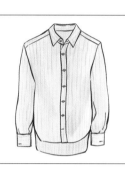

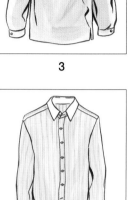

2   3

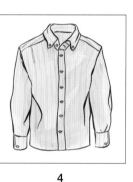

4

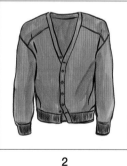

5

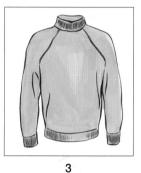

6

Sweaters

Sweaters are a great alternative to jackets for a casual look.

1 Crew neck. Not for those with a short neck.
2 Cardigan. Good for Rectangle and Rounded.
3 Roll-neck sweater with raglan sleeves (not for rounded shoulders). Good for average to long necks.
4 Chunky. Good for the Rectangle.
5 Sleeveless V-neck.
6 V-neck.

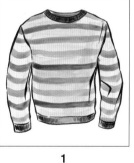

1

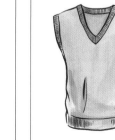

2

3

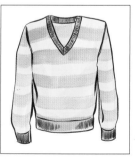

4   5   6

Tops

1 Hooded top. Great for Naturals and those who like a relaxed look.
2 Waistcoat (vest). Can add colour and flair for Dramatics and Creatives.
3 Loose t-shirt.
4 Fitted T-shirt, v-neck. Good for the Inverted triangle and Rectangle.
5 Rugby shirt. Good for Inverted triangles and Rectangles; also for Rounded in plain colours.
6 Polo shirt. Great alternative to a casual shirt.

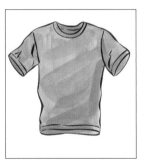

1

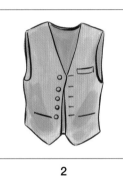

2

3

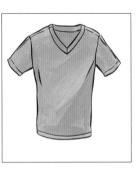

4

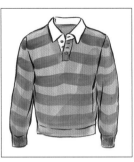

5

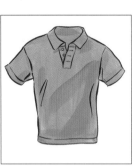

6

Trousers

1 Chinos.
2 Cargos. Good if you have long legs.
3 Drawstrings. Good for a fluctuating waist and for comfort.
4 Pleated front. Good for the Rounded figure.
5 Slim leg. Will give the illusion of longer legs.
6 Shorts. Make sure they finish at a narrow point of your leg.

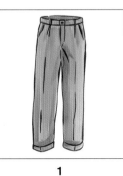

1

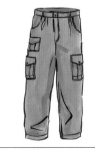

2

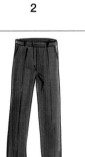

3

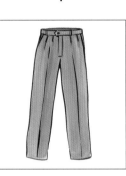

4

5

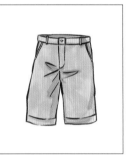

6

Jackets

1 Blouson. Excellent for Rounded figures.
2 Denim. Suits the Inverted triangle and Rectangle.
3 Sports jacket.
4 Leather jacket. Good for the Inverted triangle and Rectangle.
5 Wax.
6 Fleece. Suited to the Rectangle and Rounded.

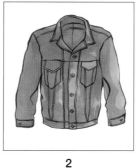 1

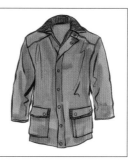 2

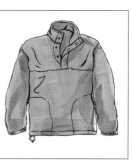 3

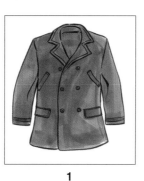 4

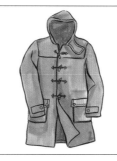 5

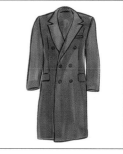 6

Coats

1 Pea coat. For the Inverted triangle and Rectangle.
2 Duffle.
3 Double-breasted. For the Inverted triangle and Rectangle.
4 Crombie.
5 Belted trench.
6 Raincoat.

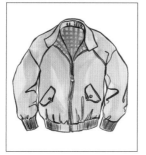 1

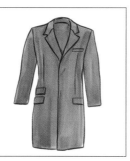 2

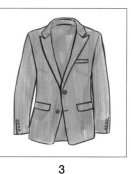 3

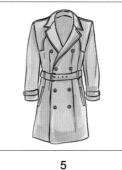 4

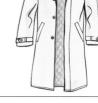 5

6

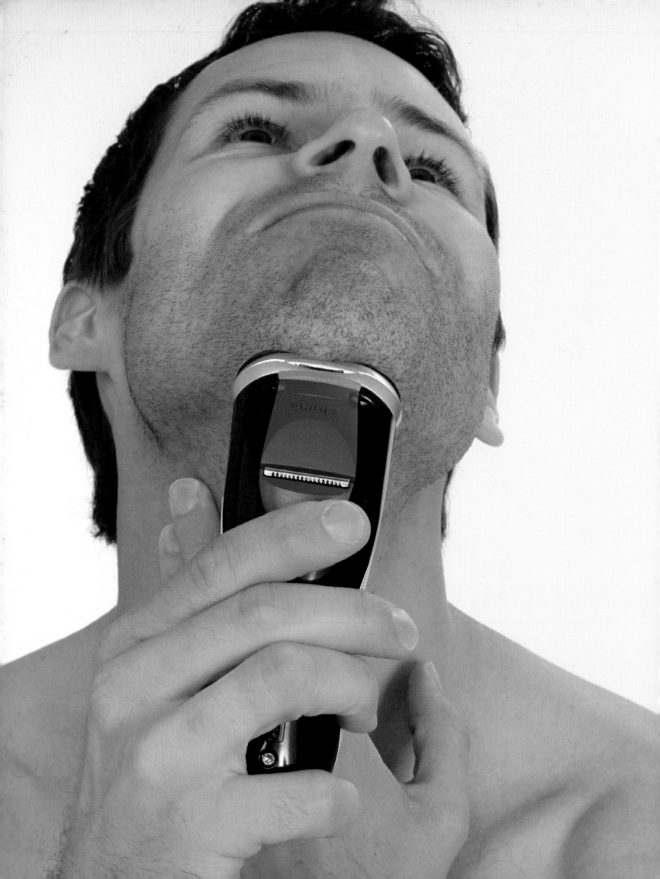

7

face facts

What's your face shape?

Now that you have established which colours and style of clothes you should be wearing, you need to make sure you choose the right hairstyle and spectacles, if you wear them. These depend very much on the shape of your face, so decide which of the following face shapes best describes you.

Chiselled face

You have an angled face with prominent cheekbones and forehead, and a square jaw.

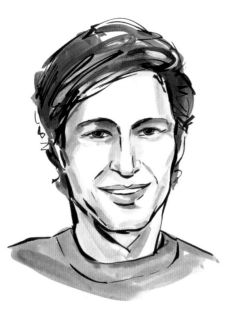

Your best hairstyles
A full head of hair Most hairstyles suit you but avoid a short brush cut (where hair is cut in a straight line at the crown 'like a brush'), which will only sharpen the angles further.
Thinning hair Keep your hair short and flat on top with graduated layers at the sides.

The spectacles for you...
Avoid very sharp angled or completely rounded frames.

Long face

You have a narrow face, which is longer than it is wide, often with a long forehead, nose and chin.

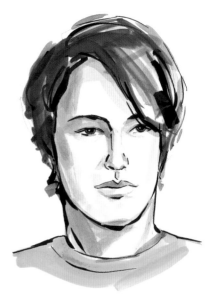

Your best hairstyles
A full head of hair A side parting, or no parting at all is best for you. Combing your hair forward will shorten the forehead, while graduating layers at the side will give width.
Thinning hair Have your hair cut to a grade 2 or 3 on top, and 4 at the sides.

The spectacles for you...
You need to give your face width, so spectacles that extend beyond your face are good for you.

Head shape

The head shape is the shape of your skull as seen from the side. A perfectly shaped skull will be slightly rounded at the back. If the back of your head appears flat, you need to create some roundness by having a graduated hairstyle, which is longer and thicker at the crown, thinning and shortening towards the nape of the neck. Always ask your hairdresser for advice.

Round face

You have full cheeks and a rounded jaw line, and may well have a double chin.

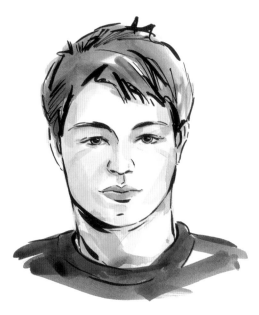

Your best hairstyles
A full head of hair You need to have the same length hair all over. If you have a parting make sure it is not centred.
Thinning hair Have your hair cut to a grade 2 or 3 all over.

The spectacles for you...
You have the choice of going frameless or having slightly rectangular frames.

Square face

You have a face where the width and length are the same. You have a square jaw line and flat forehead.

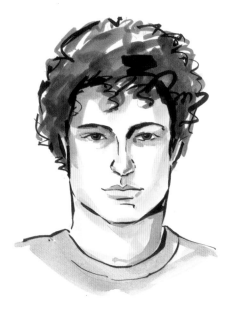

Your best hairstyles
A full head of hair Your hair needs to be longer on top with some height if possible – spiky hairstyles are good. Keep it short at the sides and avoid a sharp edge at the crown.
Thinning hair Have your hair cut to a grade 3 or 4 on top, and 2 at the sides.

The spectacles for you...
You need to give some soft angles to your face, so try oval-shaped frames.

Facial hair

Many men are unused to spending time and energy grooming themselves, but an unruly beard or moustache or wild-looking eyebrows will completely destroy an otherwise well-groomed look. If you don't feel confident about looking after any of these, seek professional advice from your hairdresser/barber.

Beards and moustaches

Facial hair can be used either for balancing your facial proportions, or as part of individualizing your look. Fashion often determines the shape and fullness of beards and moustaches. Some men wear them because of religious beliefs, others because their skin is intolerant to shaving. The size of sideburns is often fashion-led but they can help to shape your face, accentuating cheekbones, for example.

Chin

If you have a small chin, consider growing a small goatee beard to enhance the length of your chin. If, on the other hand, you have a prominent chin, consider sporting a well-trimmed beard that covers the whole of your chin and jaw. Keep your beard neatly trimmed and conditioned, following a regular care routine. A scruffy beard projects the wrong image.

Mouth

If you have a thin upper lip, consider growing a moustache or a full goatee beard. A good barber will be able to style a beard to suit your requirements.

Nasal and ear hair

Remove any visible nasal or ear hair with tweezers or small specialized clippers. Battery-powered nasal-hair trimmers are also available, which are quick if not necessarily painless!

Eyebrows

Men don't normally shape their eyebrows in the way that women do, but that doesn't mean that they can ignore this area of their face. There are two definite things to avoid:

✗ The unibrow is where your eyebrows meet in the middle. Use tweezers to remove enough of the offending hair so as to give yourself two distinct eyebrows.

✗ Long straggly hair needs to be removed with tweezers or ask your hairdresser/barber to trim your eyebrows.

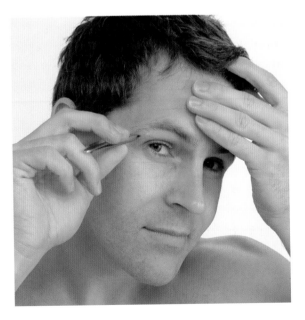

Haircare

Traditionally, men visited their barber for a 'short back and sides' and that was the end of it. Nowadays, with so many male fashion icons, increasing numbers of men are venturing down the path of looking at hair products and hair care; some even dream the dream of welcoming back a disappearing hairline.

Colour

When men's hair turns grey, it tends to give them a look of elegance and sophistication. Don't fight it. Flecks of grey are known as 'salt and pepper', and look very distinguished. If you *are* considering colouring or highlighting you hair, however, it is best done by a professional. Home hair dyes for men tend to turn your hair ginger or else you end up looking as if you are wearing a helmet, as the colour is too uniform and dark. Keep highlights to a minimum, especially if your hair is short.

Styling products

Hair wax is great for adding a shine to the hair and for added styling. Gel and mousse are also useful products. Working them into the hair at the roots will give volume and height. Conversely, working it into the shaft of the hair will help to calm wild curly hair.

If you are unsure of which products to choose, ask for advice at a salon that specializes in men's grooming, and keep it simple.

More often than not, greying hair gives men a look of elegance and sophistication

Options for thinning hair

Unfortunately, there is no medical proof that by rubbing ointments into the scalp a dead hair follicle will start to produce hair again. Hair implants are an option and are improving all the time, but they are an expensive way to try to preserve your hairline.

Wigs and toupees

Wigs and toupees are best avoided if possible. Because men's hair is generally worn short, the scalp and hairline move with the facial muscles. This doesn't happen when you wear a wig or a toupee so it always looks fake. (It is not as obvious when a woman wears a wig because the hairline is generally disguised.)

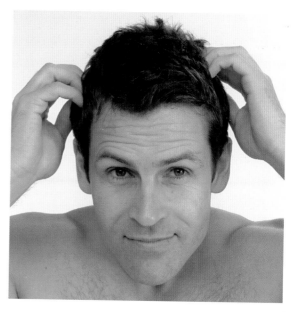

Shaving

It is personal choice as to whether you 'wet' or 'dry' shave. Whatever your preference, you need a good technique and good quality products and equipment. Wet shaving is probably better if you have a strong hair growth. Dry shaving is particularly good for those with sensitive skin or lighter beard growth.

Wet shaving

A wet shave takes time, preparation and patience. Your beard should be softened first to open up the hair follicles, either by the steam from a shower or with a hot flannel. There are also products available that will soften the beard before applying shaving cream. Always invest in good quality products – from shaving foams to razors – and you will enjoy a close, comfortable shave.

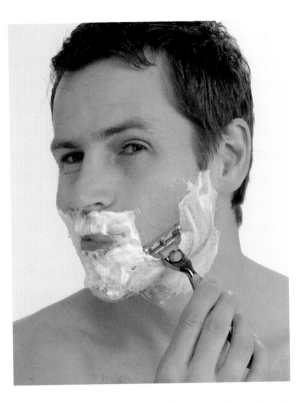

✓ Shower or bathe before shaving, or warm the face with a hot flannel.

✓ Use plenty of hot water and shave in a warm, steamy environment.

✓ If you have a strong beard, use a beard softener before shaving.

✓ Use a good quality brush with good shaving cream, soap or shaving foam.

✓ Work in a circular movement to lift the beard.

✓ Use a razor with a movable head and at least two blades, and change the blades once a week.

✓ Shave the beard with upwards strokes first. Foam up again, and then work downwards to ensure the closest possible shave.

✓ Rinse the blade frequently in hot water.

✓ Rinse your face well with cool water and gently pat dry.

A good razor – regularly updated – will ensure a perfect shave.

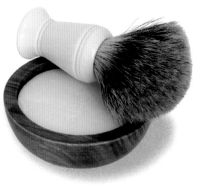

Dry shaving

There are two types of electric razors: the rotary lift and cut, and the curved side-to-side cutter. It is personal choice as to which suits you best, but choose a razor that also has a beard trimmer for your sideburns. Cordless razors are great when travelling.

✓ As for wet shaving, prepare your face by opening up the hair follicles by showering or applying a hot flannel to your skin.

✓ You can use a pre-electric shaving balm to soften the hair, but you may find this unnecessary.

✓ As you shave, lift and stretch the skin between thumb and forefinger.

✓ Electric razors can now be rinsed off after use (but do check the manufacturers' instructions).

✓ Change the cutting heads on your razor at least once a year.

After shaving care

✓ A good wet shave exfoliates (removes the dead skin cells that collect on the surface of the skin) and cleanses the skin, leaving smooth new skin and a healthy clean appearance.

✓ If you dry shave you should use a facial scrub, or exfoliator (see page 152), every other day to remove dead skin cells from the surface of the skin.

✓ Newly exfoliated skin needs to be protected from the elements, so use an after-shaving moisturizer, preferably with sun filters.

✓ Products containing alcohol should not be applied to the skin directly after shaving, whether wet or dry, as this may inflame the skin and cause dryness. Choose a balm instead but check first that it will not irritate your skin.

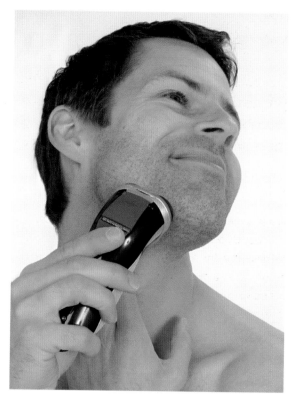

An electric razor is a good idea if you travel a lot or need a clean-shaven face at the end of the day.

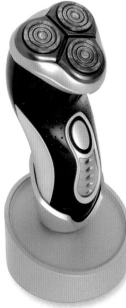

Facial skincare

The skin is the largest organ in the body and is constantly renewing itself. Imagine your skin as an escalator, with new plump skin cells being formed at the bottom and, as they rise to the top, they lose their moisture, dry up and eventually flake off. This process takes approximately 23–28 days – the older you get, the slower the process.

Cleansing, exfoliating and toning

By removing the dead skin cells regularly, the newer and plumper cells give the skin the appearance of a healthier glow. Although shaving will remove some of the dead skin cells you obviously don't shave the whole of your face. Over the past decade or so, men's grooming products have become more sophisticated and you should be able to find one to suit you.

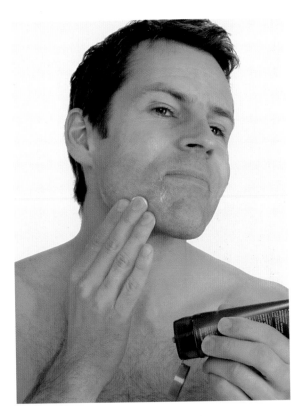

Foreheads and noses are normally the oiliest part of the face and need some form of cleansing. For most men the ideal solution is to use a facial scrub when showering. Designed to remove dead skin cells and exfoliate the skin, gentle facial scrubs can be used daily while others are best as a weekly treat. Read the manufacturer's instructions on how best to use them as they all vary depending on the formulation. After use ensure that you completely rinse the scrub off your face before drying.

If you have a sensitive skin a proprietary cream cleanser will give you the same results, but you will need to use a toner afterwards to ensure that all the cream cleanser is effectively removed.

Moisturizing

Skin cells are full of the body's natural moisture but central heating, air conditioning and even the heater in your car can dry out your skin, and lead to premature ageing. Using a moisturizer helps trap the skin's natural moisture for longer. By having a healthy outer layer of skin, the deeper levels of your skin are better protected. Many moisturizers contain some form of filter to protect your skin from the damaging effects of the sun, and also help protect it against air pollutants.

When applying moisturizer, massage it gently into your facial skin with your fingertips, not forgetting your neck. Applying moisturizer to elbows and knees will help to soften hard skin. If you're going bald don't forget to apply moisturizer to the top of your head, too.

Sun creams

Exposure to sunlight is very damaging to your skin and can lead to premature wrinkles. Sun creams filter out the ultraviolet rays (UVAs and UVBs) from the sun, which penetrate the skin and damage the inner layers. The longer you spend outside, the higher the protection factor of your sun cream should be.

UVA and UVB rays harm you not only on sunny days. They are there all the time, so if you are going for a long walk, playing golf, tennis or football, or working outside, don't forget to apply your sun cream. Alternatively, on a daily basis, you could use a moisturizing skincare product that contains a sunscreen. The minimum recommended sun protection factor is SPF15. Choose a product and SPF that are suited to your complexion.

Fragrance

The use of fragrance is a personal choice. Only wear a scent that you like and not because it was given to you. Never use so much of a fragrance that it lingers in the room after you leave.

Instead of using a strong scented fragrance it is better to 'layer' it. For example, make sure your shower gel, deodorant and balm are all of the same fragrance, rather than mixing them.

Aftershave

This is meant to tighten the pores that have become enlarged during a wet shave. Choose an aftershave that is alcohol-free. It should not sting the skin, but just give a gentle tingle. Apply aftershave after splashing your skin with cold water to close the pores.

Balm

This is a lotion that will also refine the pores in a gentle way. Balms are often made with natural or essential oils mixed with a soothing base, such as shea butter. Essential oils can have the additional benefits of enhancing your mood, depending on their aromatherapy qualities.

Eau de toilette

This is the modern man's equivalent to perfume. For best results, this should be applied to the pulse points on the inside of the wrists and on the sides of the neck.

The longer you spend outside, the higher the protection factor of your sun cream.

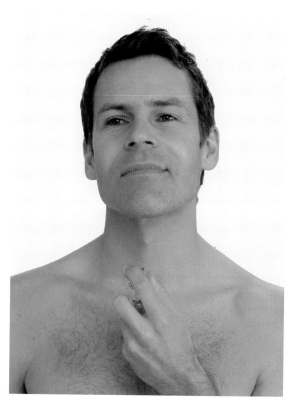

From top to toe

Male grooming is not just about hair and facial skincare – the whole body needs looking after, from top to toe. Make sure you allow yourself enough time on a weekly basis for some body maintenance – there's no reason why body pampering should be a female-only domain.

A winning smile

When you meet someone for the first time and shake their hand, not only are they looking into your eyes, they are also looking at your mouth and hence your teeth. A winning smile is an important part of any person's image. How you achieve this depends on the state of your teeth. Not everyone has picture-perfect teeth, but it is possible to keep both your teeth and gums healthy and clean.

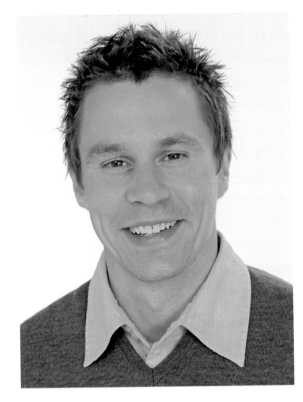

✓ Visit your dentist once a year for a check-up and undergo any necessary treatment.

✓ Visit your hygienist at least twice a year to ensure your teeth and gums stay healthy, and your breath is fresh.

✓ Floss daily and follow your hygienist's advice on how to maintain a healthy mouth.

✓ For discoloured teeth, consider bleaching them. This can be done at home with a special treatment available from your dentist. Alternatively, specialist treatment such as capping, crowning or porcelain veneers are available at a cost.

✓ Sometimes orthodontic treatment is the only way to correct your teeth. Although expensive, this is becoming more popular with adults.

Fresh breath is essential in all social situations, whether at work or at play. If you've had a heavy business lunch, or just a long day at the office, keep some mouthwash, a toothbrush and toothpaste in your drawer or bag, for an instant freshen-up.

Keep your teeth healthy as a winning smile is an important part of your well-groomed image.

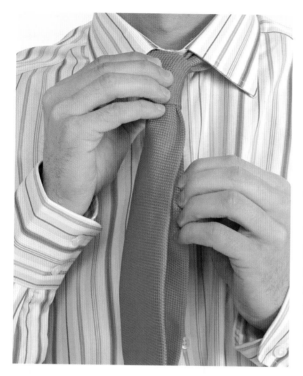

Keep your nails clean and neatly trimmed to ensure a groomed handshake.

A groomed handshake

Your hands reflect your lifestyle. Whatever that lifestyle is, some care is needed to maintain well-groomed hands and nails. Treat yourself to a professional manicure and then maintain the shape yourself with a regular handcare routine.

✓ Keep your nails short and clean.

✓ Cuticles need to be pushed back to prevent them becoming split and painful. Do this after bathing when the cuticles are soft, using either the thumb of the opposite hand or a specialized rubber-tipped hoofer. Be careful not to damage the nail bed.

✓ Have regular manicures if your hands are on show and it is important that they look good. A manicure is especially important if you are a nail biter – every time you're tempted to put your fingers in your mouth, remember how much you spent on your hands.

✓ If you have dry and sore hands, use a non-perfumed hand cream.

✓ To soften calluses and hard skin, use a pumice stone or a home-made scrub made of sea salt and lemon juice.

Those feet are made for walking

Your feet are probably the hardest working part of your body yet they are often neglected. You should look after them – just think of what they do for you in the confines of your shoes. A little TLC will go along way to putting a spring in your step. If you have any problems with your feet, make an appointment to see a chiropodist or podiatrist.

✓ Make sure you wear the correct size shoes.

✓ Wear socks made of breathable material like cotton or wool and make sure they are roomy enough so that your toes can move freely.

✓ Trim your toe nails regularly and avoid leaving sharp corners to prevent ingrowing toe nails.

✓ Use a pumice stone or loofah to remove hard skin.

✓ After showering or bathing, make sure you dry them well, particularly in between the toes.

✓ Remember that if you catch a verruca, it won't go away on its own and it will need to be treated.

✓ Some men suffer from yeast infections of the nail bed – see a chiropodist or your doctor for correct diagnosis and treatment.

✓ Treat yourself to a pedicure once in a while.

✓ Keep your feet and toe nails clean and trimmed if wearing sandals in the summer.

The age factor

Having taken in all the advice in the previous pages of this book, you now need to bring it all together to create the image that matters. Your age is a strong determining factor of what is right and what is wrong for you. As you mature, you will need to adapt your style and perhaps be aware that your colours may change, too.

In your 20s

✓ You are establishing your identity.

✓ Experiment with colours and styles that suit you and your lifestyle.

✓ Learn to care and look after your clothes.

✓ If you are on a limited budget, buy sensibly and look at the suggested core wardrobe (see pages 130–131).

✓ Keep up your chosen sports.

✗ Avoid excesses in alcohol, food and nicotine.

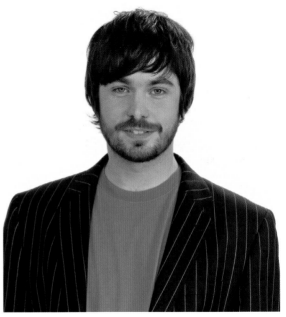

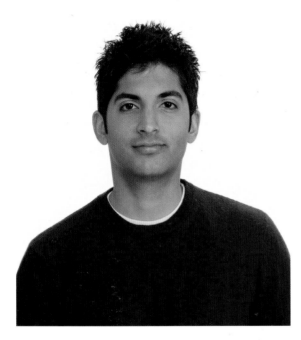

In your 30s

✓ You have your preferred style and know where you like to shop.

✓ Leave the popular icon image behind. Be your own man.

✓ Don't let other demands on your budget stop you from investing in your wardrobe – a good quality suit will adapt to both work and social occasions.

✓ Now is the time to remember to make those hygienist appointments.

✓ Review your hairstyle, particularly if your hair is thinning.

✓ Despite a busy lifestyle, try to avoid snacking.

In your 40s

✓ Keep looking current – which doesn't mean dressing like a teenager.

✓ Try new colours and styles in your current size.

✓ If you have given up on skincare, now is the time to resume it for a healthy-looking complexion.

✓ Sun protection is a must.

✓ Consult a stylist to ensure your hairstyle is appropriate for the amount of hair that you have, and to update your look.

✓ Watch your waistline and where your trousers are sitting.

✓ Ensure you have regular health checks.

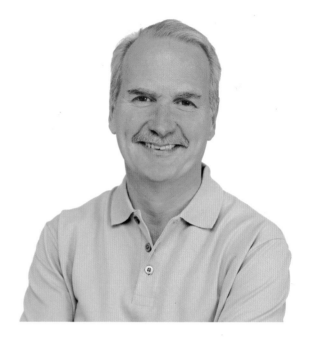

In your 50s and thereafter

✓ Dress for comfort while staying current.

✓ Go for a low-maintenance easy-care wardrobe.

✓ Shop regularly even if your clothes are not worn out.

✓ Only wear clothes that you like and that suit your colouring and build.

✓ Exercise both the body and the mind daily.

✓ Treat yourself to a little luxury now and then.

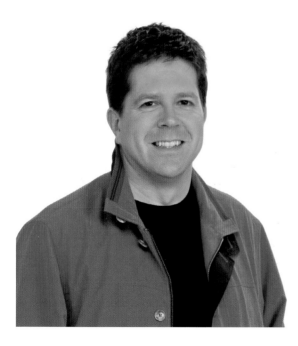

Index

Acknowledgements

When it comes to men, we come from different worlds. Pat likes them more casual and relaxed, whilst Veronique prefers them in suits and dapper. This book was written with all types of men in mind.

The whole Hamlyn team were as supportive as ever, from editing to design. Thank you to all involved in putting **Colour Me Confident's** little brother to bed.

Many thanks to our willing models who did not dare to disagree with us once! Cliff Bashforth, Alan Bryon, Tim Doran, Steven Gauge, Mark Holland, Charlie McArdle, Steve Ravenscroft, Ian Reilly, Bob Trusty, Mark Watson, Shaun Williams and Jack Zouain were real stars, gracious at all times and some of them are even wearing their own clothes.

Thank you to Philip Child of W.G. Child & Sons, bespoke tailors since 1890, who spent time with us to answer the detailed sartorial questions we presented him with.

Huge thank yous to Audrey Hanna who charmed and coordinated our models and held our hands on many occasions (she's on p 93), and to Rosalie Poels who shopped 'til she dropped to make sure we had all the right clothes for our models. Thank you for all your support, we could not have done it without you.

Thank you to all the PRs who so kindly arranged for us to use their clothes (see list below).

Thank you to Chris Scarles, our MD, who so appropriately commented on our first draft and who so willingly modelled too. He was our inspiration!

Most of what we know about men comes from our respective husbands and sons (and son-in-law for Pat) who we bore in mind at every page. They all had to read and comment on the first draft. Thank you to Jim Henshaw and John Henderson for letting us loose in their wardrobes; whilst Tom Henderson's own walk-in closet provided most of the 'funky' pieces for the photoshoot.

And finally, a big thank you to each other too!

Pat Henshaw and Veronique Henderson

Clothes acknowledgements:

Austin Reed www.austinreed.co.uk
Burton www.burton.co.uk
Dormeuil www.dormeuil.com
Esprit www.esprit.com
Haines & Bonner www.haines-bonner.co.uk
Haggar +44 (0)20 7297 6890
Jaeger www.jaeger.co.uk
Lacoste www.lacoste.com
Pierre Cardin +44 (0)1582 509 882
Thomas Pink www.thomaspink.co.uk

For more information on services, products and how to become a consultant contact **colour me beautiful**:

UK and Headquarters for Europe, Africa and the Middle East
66 The Business Centre, 15–17 Ingate Place, London SW8 3NS
www.colourmebeautiful.co.uk and www.cmb.co.uk
info@cmb.co.uk
t: +44 (0)20 7627 5211
f: +44 (0)20 7627 5680

Americas and Australasia www.colormebeautiful.com
T: (001) 1-800-606 3435
Germany, Netherlands, Austria, Belgium & Switzerland
www.colourmebeautiful.nu
France, Italy, Russia www.colourmebeautiful.com
China www.qixincolor.com
Ireland www.cmb-ireland.ie
Hong Kong www.colormebeautiful.hk
Finland colormebeautiful@kolumbi.fi
Norway & Denmark www.colormebeautiful.no
Slovenia www.cmb.si
South Africa www.colormebeautiful.co.za
Spain www.cmb-asesoresdeimagen.com
Sweden www.colormebeautiful.se

Picture Acknowledgements

Special photography: Octopus Publishing Group Limited/Mike Prior.

Corbis UK Ltd/Rufus F Folkks 20 top right, 20 bottom centre, 34 bottom right, 38 bottom, 86; /Mitchell Gerber 20 bottom left, 26 bottom; /Tim Graham 20 top centre, 30 bottom, 91 left; /Frank Trapper 20 top left, 22 bottom, 91 right. **Getty Images**/Chris Jackson 21 right; /Pierre Philippe Marcou 78; /Kevin Winter 80. **Rex Features** 76; /AGF 20 bottom right, 42 bottom; /Stuart Atkins 82; /Mark Campbell 84; /Nils Jorgensen 21 left.

For hamlyn

Executive Editor Sarah Ford
Editor Charlotte Macey
Creative Director Geoff Fennell
Designer 'ome design
Illustrator Kevin Jones Associates
Senior Production Controller Martin Croshaw
Picture Researcher Emma O'Neill